PERFECT EYES WITHOUT GLASSES

A GUIDE TO NATURAL VISION IMPROVEMENT

GEOFFREY ZACHARY

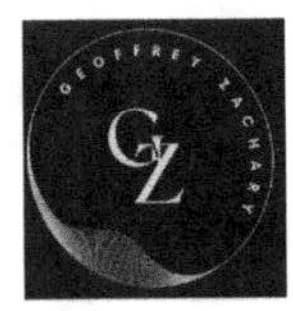

CONTENTS

Perfect Sight Without Glasses:

A Guide to Natural Vision Improvement

Introduction

In the corridors of human history, our understanding of eyesight has undergone numerous metamorphoses. From the ancient civilizations that believed in spiritual reasons for vision loss to the current digital era, where screens threaten to strain our eyes, the journey of comprehending eyesight has been nothing short of fascinating.

Historically, eyesight was often regarded as a mystical phenomenon. The ancient Egyptians believed that the eye was a representation of the Udjat or the 'Eye of Horus', symbolizing protection and good health. They didn't comprehend refractive errors, but they recognized the significance of protecting one's eyesight.

By the time of the ancient Greeks and Romans, there was a shift towards a more clinical understanding of the eyes. Great thinkers like Hippocrates and Galen started dissecting eyes, laying the groundwork for future anatomical studies. However, the basic premise was simple: the eye captures what we see and sends it to the brain. The specifics, especially concerning vision problems, remained largely misunderstood.

Fast forward to the Middle Ages and the Renaissance, where eyeglasses made their historical debut. The invention of the first wearable glasses, which date back to the end of the 13th century in Italy, marked a pivotal shift. No longer was poor eyesight just a lamentable fate; it could be corrected. As revolutionary as this was, it also led to the onset of numerous misconceptions about vision. The most persistent of these is the idea that once your vision starts deteriorating, the only solution is a stronger prescription.

With time, as science and technology advanced, so did our understanding of the eyes. By the 19th and 20th centuries, optometry had emerged as a dedicated field of medicine. Vision problems were classified, diagnosed, and treated with an array of lenses and, eventually, surgeries. Yet, alongside these advancements arose a belief that glasses or surgical interventions were the only pathways to clear vision.

This is where the essence of our guide comes into focus. Natural vision improvement is not a new concept, but for many, it remains an unexplored territory. Over the past century, researchers and holistic health practitioners alike have delved into methods that promise better vision without the aid of glasses or surgery. From the renowned Bates Method to exercises that train the eye muscles, these techniques have offered hope to countless individuals.

So, is natural vision improvement truly possible? The human body possesses a remarkable capacity for healing and adaptation. Just as a broken bone can mend itself or the brain can rewire its connections following an injury, the eyes too have the potential for improvement. The key lies in understanding that vision isn't solely dependent on the eyes' anatomical structure, but also on the brain, the way we use our eyes, and our overall well-being.

This book endeavours to provide a holistic view of eyesight, breaking down age-old myths and guiding you towards a clearer vision, both literally and metaphorically. It's a journey that will challenge widely held beliefs, but with an open mind, it's a journey that promises clarity, understanding, and a fresh perspective on the wonders of vision.

As you navigate the chapters ahead, remember that the quest for perfect sight is not just about seeing the world with clarity but understanding our place within it. It's about reclaiming a facet of our health that many of us have taken for granted and recognizing that, sometimes, the answers aren't found in a prescription but within ourselves and the world around us. Welcome to a transformative exploration of sight, light, and perception. Welcome to "Perfect Sight Without Glasses."

Part I: Understanding Eyesight

CHAPTER 1: THE MECHANICS OF VISION

Vision, at its most basic level, is light interacting with our eyes. Yet, the processes that transform light waves into images in our minds are incredibly intricate. This chapter is dedicated to understanding the core mechanics of vision, from the journey of a photon as it enters our eye to the electrical impulses that let us "see" in our brain.

1. How the Eye Captures Light: The Cornea and the Lens

Our eyes are often compared to cameras, and there's an excellent reason for this analogy. Imagine the cornea as the camera's outer lens. This transparent layer is responsible for allowing light to enter the eye. Its curved shape helps bend or 'refract' this light, directing it towards the lens.

Just behind the cornea lies the iris, the coloured part of our eyes, which can expand or contract to control the amount of light entering the eye. The black circle in the middle of the iris is the pupil, a sort of 'gateway' for light.

Now, once light passes through the pupil, it encounters the eye's natural lens. This lens, unlike the fixed lens of a camera, can change shape. It can become flatter or rounder, adjusting the direction of the incoming light to ensure that it's focused precisely onto the retina, a process known as accommodation.

2. Transforming Light into Images: The Role of the Retina

The retina is a thin layer of tissue lining the back of the eye. Think of it as a cinema screen, but instead of displaying movies, it receives the focused light from the lens. Embedded within the retina are millions of photoreceptor cells – rods and cones. These cells are sensitive to light and play a fundamental role in our vision.

Rods handle low-light conditions and peripheral vision. They don't differentiate colours but are extremely sensitive, allowing us to see even when it's quite dark. Cones, on the other hand, operate in well-lit conditions and enable us to perceive colour. Humans have three types of cones, each sensitive to a specific range of light wavelengths – red, green, or blue. Together, they enable us to experience the full spectrum of colours.

When light strikes these photoreceptors, a remarkable transformation occurs. The energy from the light triggers a chemical reaction, converting it into an electrical signal.

3. The Information Superhighway: The Optic Nerve

The optic nerve is the bridge between the eye and the brain. This bundle of over a million nerve fibres transmits the electrical signals from the retina to the brain. Each fibre carries a fragment of the visual puzzle, a minute detail of the overall picture.

Before the optic nerve exits the eye, the nerve fibres gather at a point on the retina called the optic disc. Interestingly, this area lacks photoreceptors, leading to what we commonly refer to as the 'blind spot'. However, our brain adeptly fills in this gap, ensuring we perceive a continuous image.

4. Decoding Light: The Brain's Role in Vision

While our eyes capture and convert light, it's our brain that 'sees'. The electrical signals from the optic nerve travel to the brain's visual cortex, located at the back of the head. Here, these signals are processed, interpreted, and combined with our other senses to produce the rich tapestry of vision we experience.

The visual cortex decodes factors like shape, colour, depth, and movement, harmonizing them into a coherent, dynamic image. This entire process, from light entering our eyes to our conscious recognition of an image, happens almost instantaneously, showcasing the incredible efficiency and complexity of our visual system.

In conclusion, understanding the mechanics of vision underscores the miraculous nature of our eyesight. The intricate coordination between the eye's various components and our brain's processing power is a testament to the marvel of evolution and biology. Recognizing this complexity not only fosters a deeper appreciation for our sight but also highlights the potential for natural interventions to harness the eye's innate adaptability. As we delve deeper into the world of natural vision improvement, this foundational knowledge will serve as our guiding light.

CHAPTER 2: COMMON VISION PROBLEMS

In understanding vision, it's crucial to comprehend not only the mechanics of how we see but also the common issues that can impede our sight. This chapter delves into some of the most prevalent vision problems: myopia, hyperopia, astigmatism, and presbyopia. By demystifying these conditions, we can better appreciate the steps toward natural vision improvement.

**1. Myopia (Near-sightedness) **

*What it is: * Myopia, commonly referred to as near-sightedness, is a refractive error where distant objects appear blurred while close objects can be seen clearly. This is due to the eye's shape being slightly elongated, causing light to focus in front of the retina instead of directly on it.

*Causes and considerations: * The exact cause of myopia is still debated, but it's believed to be a mix of genetic and environmental factors. Extended close-up work, like reading or screen time, has been identified as a potential contributor. Urbanization and reduced time spent outdoors have also been linked to rising rates of myopia worldwide.

2. Hyperopia (Farsightedness)

*What it is: * The inverse of myopia, hyperopia or farsightedness, means distant objects can be seen more clearly than those close up. This occurs when the eye is slightly shorter than average, causing light to focus behind the retina.

*Causes and considerations: * Hyperopia can be congenital, meaning some people are born with it. While many babies are born farsighted, they often outgrow the condition as their eyes grow and lengthen. However, some retain it into adulthood. As with myopia, both genetic and environmental factors can contribute.

3. Astigmatism

*What it is: * Astigmatism arises when the cornea, instead of being round, is shaped more like an American football. This irregular shape results in light focusing on multiple points around the retina, rather than a single point. It can cause blurred or distorted vision at any distance.

*Causes and considerations: * Most people have some degree of astigmatism, and it often occurs alongside myopia or hyperopia. It's believed to be largely hereditary. Regular eye exams are crucial as astigmatism can change over time or remain stable.

4. Presbyopia

*What it is: * Unlike the other conditions discussed, presbyopia isn't a refractive error but an age-related condition. As we age, the eye's lens becomes less flexible, making it harder to focus on close objects. This is why many older adults need reading glasses.

*Causes and considerations: * Presbyopia is a natural part of the aging process. Around the age of 40, many begin to notice it's harder to read small print or do close-up tasks. While it's inevitable, regular eye exams can help monitor its progression and offer solutions to manage it.

The Bigger Picture

While these common vision problems might seem distinct, they share a crucial commonality: they all result from the eye's inability to focus light precisely on the retina. The causes and manifestations might differ, but the core issue is how light interacts with our eyes.

Many conventional treatments for these conditions involve corrective lenses or surgical interventions. These solutions undoubtedly offer clearer vision, but they address the symptoms without necessarily considering the root causes or the holistic health of the eye.

Furthermore, our modern lifestyles—marked by extended screen time, artificial lighting, and reduced outdoor activities—play a pivotal role in our eye health. As we journey further into natural vision improvement, understanding these foundational issues provides a basis for holistic strategies that consider the entire well-being of the eyes and the individual.

In subsequent chapters, we'll explore not just how these conditions arise, but how lifestyle modifications, exercises, and a deeper comprehension of eye health can pave the way for better sight, without always resorting to glasses.

CHAPTER 3. THE CAUSES OF VISION IMPAIRMENTS

Our eyes, often referred to as the windows to our souls, are complex and delicate organs, responsible for bringing the visual world into sharp focus. It's a marvel when you think about the multitude of factors that must come together to provide you with clear vision. However, many of us, at some point in our lives, experience vision impairments. Understanding the root causes can be the first step in addressing and potentially reversing these conditions.

Environmental Factors

*1. Prolonged Screen Time: * With the digital age, many of us spend hours glued to screens - be it computers, smartphones, or television. This can lead to digital eye strain. The blue light emitted by screens can be harmful in large doses, causing fatigue, dry eyes, and potentially leading to more serious conditions over time.

*2. UV Exposure: * Sunlight contains ultraviolet (UV) rays which can be harmful to the eyes, leading to conditions like cataracts or macular degeneration. Not wearing protective eyewear, like sunglasses with UV protection, can expose the eyes to this risk.

*3. Pollution: * Air pollution can cause irritation, dryness, and allergies, which can all impact vision if left untreated.

Particulate matter and chemicals in the air can irritate the eye's surface.

Genetic Factors

*1. Heredity: * Just as we inherit physical traits like the colour of our hair or height from our parents, we can also inherit the propensity for certain eye conditions. Conditions like myopia (short-sightedness), hyperopia (farsightedness), and astigmatism can run in families.

*2. Congenital Issues: * Some vision problems are present at birth. Conditions like congenital cataracts or amblyopia (lazy eye) might be due to genetic mutations or complications during pregnancy.

Lifestyle Factors

*1. Diet and Nutrition: * Our eyes, like the rest of our body, require specific nutrients to function optimally. A diet lacking in vitamins like C and E, minerals like zinc, and other nutrients like omega-3 fatty acids can impact eye health, leading to conditions like macular degeneration.

*2. Smoking: * It's well known that smoking is detrimental to overall health, but it can also significantly affect vision. Smoking increases the risk of cataracts, damages the optic nerve, and can lead to age-related macular degeneration.

*3. Lack of Physical Exercise: * Regular physical activity can reduce the risk of vision problems. Exercise improves blood circulation, ensuring adequate oxygen reaches the eyes and aids in the removal of toxins.

*4. Improper Reading Habits: * Reading in poor light or holding reading materials too close can strain the eyes, potentially leading to myopia in younger individuals.

*5. Alcohol Consumption: * Excessive drinking can lead to optic neuropathy, a condition that can harm the optic nerve, causing vision loss.

Understanding these causes is vital. If you recognize certain behaviours or factors in your life that might be detrimental to your vision, you can start to make changes. For instance, ensuring you take regular breaks if you work at a computer, or incorporating nutrient-rich foods into your diet, can have profound effects on your visual health.

Moreover, acknowledging genetic factors can help you be more proactive. If your family has a history of a particular eye condition, regular check-ups and early intervention can make all the difference.

It's also essential to remember that our eyes don't operate in isolation. They are an integral part of our body, and their health often mirrors our overall well-being. Factors that generally benefit our health—like a balanced diet, physical activity, and refraining from smoking or excessive alcohol consumption— not only benefit our heart, lungs, and muscles, but our eyes as well.

In the subsequent chapters, we will delve deeper into practices and remedies to counteract these challenges. But the first step in any journey of improvement is understanding the root cause, and with eyes, it's no different. By appreciating the multitude of factors that can impair our vision, we set the stage for strategies to achieve perfect sight without glasses.

CHAPTER 4. DEBUNKING EYEGLASSES MYTHS

Eyeglasses: they've been around for centuries, aiding countless individuals in seeing the world more clearly. However, along with their widespread use has come a slew of myths and misconceptions. In this chapter, we'll tackle one of the most prominent myths surrounding eyeglasses: Do they actually worsen eyesight over time?

Understanding the Purpose of Glasses

To debunk this myth, it's essential first to understand the purpose of eyeglasses. Eyeglasses are corrective devices that compensate for the eye's inability to focus light directly onto the retina. They don't "cure" vision problems but adjust the light entering the eye so that images appear clear.

Whether it's for near-sightedness (myopia), farsightedness (hyperopia), astigmatism, or presbyopia, glasses modify the light's path to ensure it focuses correctly, offering a clearer view of the world.

**Do Glasses Worsen Eyesight? **

*The Myth: * A common belief is that once you start wearing glasses, your eyes become "dependent" on them, causing your vision to deteriorate faster than it would if you weren't wearing them.

*The Reality: * This notion, though widespread, is largely a misconception. When people start wearing glasses, they become accustomed to a clearer and sharper world. Without glasses, they're then more acutely aware of their uncorrected vision, leading to the perception that their eyesight has worsened. In reality, the vision would likely have deteriorated at the same rate, glasses or no glasses.

Another aspect to consider is the natural progression of eye conditions. For example, myopia in children and teenagers often progresses as they grow, irrespective of whether they wear glasses. Thus, the need for a stronger prescription over time is not necessarily due to the glasses themselves but rather the natural course of the condition.

Adapting to Clarity

When someone first starts wearing glasses, especially after a prolonged period of blurry vision, the sudden clarity can be startling. It's like upgrading from a low-resolution video to high definition instantly. This sudden shift might be interpreted as dependency, but it's merely an appreciation of clearer vision. Over time, this becomes the new normal, making it harder to revert to a blurrier state.

Potential Pitfalls

While glasses don't cause vision to deteriorate, improper or outdated prescriptions can lead to issues. Wearing glasses that aren't suited to your current vision needs can cause eyestrain, headaches, and discomfort. This emphasizes the importance of regular eye exams to ensure your prescription matches your needs.

Benefits Beyond Correction

Apart from vision correction, glasses can offer protection. They shield the eyes from dust and debris, and with the right coatings, they can protect against harmful UV rays and reduce glare.

Natural Vision Improvement and Glasses

Does this mean those on a journey of natural vision improvement should shun glasses? Not necessarily. While the goal might be to reduce dependency on them, glasses can be a valuable tool. They ensure safety while driving or performing tasks that require precise vision. As natural vision techniques are employed and vision improves, prescriptions can be adjusted.

Conclusion

The belief that glasses worsen eyesight is rooted in misunderstandings and the stark difference between corrected and uncorrected vision. Glasses are tools designed to provide clarity, and they don't intrinsically degrade eyesight. While the journey to perfect sight without glasses is commendable and achievable, it's essential to approach it with a balanced perspective. Embrace the clarity that glasses provide, even as you work holistically to nurture and improve your innate vision.

Part II: Techniques for Natural Vision Improvement

CHAPTER 5: THE BATES METHOD

One of the most famous approaches to natural vision improvement is the Bates Method. To grasp its significance and practices, it's essential to delve into its history, principles, and the transformative impact it has had on many individuals worldwide.

1. Historical Context

Dr. William Horatio Bates, an American ophthalmologist in the early 20th century, introduced the Bates Method. Despite the significant medical advances of his time, Bates grew sceptical about the then-prevailing understanding of refractive errors. He was particularly concerned about the over-reliance on glasses, which he believed merely acted as a crutch rather than a cure.

Over his extensive career, he observed anomalies in vision that couldn't be explained by the predominant theories. For instance, he noticed that some people's vision would fluctuate, challenging the idea that refractive errors were static and unchangeable.

Driven by these observations, Bates embarked on exhaustive research and experimentation. His findings culminated in the development of a series of exercises and practices aimed at improving vision naturally, without the need for corrective lenses.

2. Principles of the Bates Method

The Bates Method revolves around a few core principles:

- **Relaxation is Crucial: ** Dr. Bates postulated that strain, whether mental or physical, is the primary cause of vision problems. By relieving this strain, one could improve sight. Techniques like 'palming' (covering closed eyes with the hands to block out light) and deep breathing exercises are fundamental to this relaxation philosophy.

- **Use of the Eyes in Natural Conditions: ** Bates believed that natural light, especially sunlight, played a vital role in optimal eye function. The "sun treatment" involves closing the eyes, turning one's head towards the sun, and allowing the sunlight to fall on the closed lids, moving the head gently from side to side.

- **Movement and Central Fixation: ** Our eyes are designed for movement. Bates introduced exercises such as "swinging," where individuals would sway from side to side, observing objects in motion to improve flexibility and function. Central fixation, another core principle, refers to the idea that the eye sees only one small part of an object most clearly and that natural, involuntary eye movement is essential for optimal vision.

- **Visualizing and Memory: ** Bates argued that the ability to remember or visualize a scene or object in black, the blackest black imaginable, could greatly enhance clarity of vision. He introduced exercises where one would visualize familiar objects, letters, or scenes, aiming for this perfect black.

- **Avoiding Overreliance on Glasses: ** While Dr. Bates wasn't entirely against glasses, he believed they were often prescribed prematurely and used excessively. He argued that relying on them could make the eyes lazy and exacerbate vision problems.

A Holistic Take on Vision

While the Bates Method has faced both admiration and

scepticism, there's no denying the comprehensive approach it takes towards vision. Instead of merely focusing on the eyes, Bates viewed vision in the context of the whole person, encompassing mental, physical, and emotional well-being.

It's also worth noting that many users of the Bates Method have reported improvements. Anecdotal successes range from slight enhancements in clarity to individuals claiming to have discarded their glasses entirely.

A Continuing Legacy

The Bates Method continues to inspire a slew of natural vision improvement methods. While it may not be a one-size-fits-all solution, its holistic approach, emphasis on relaxation, and focus on natural conditions are undeniably valuable perspectives in the realm of eye care.

In subsequent chapters, we will delve into specific exercises from the Bates Method and other natural vision practices, offering readers a chance to experiment and discern what might work best for their unique needs.

As with any method or technique, it's essential to approach it with an open yet discerning mind, being open to potential benefits but also considering the broader context of one's overall health and well-being.

CHAPTER 6: PALMING

Imagine a technique so simple yet profoundly impactful that it not only relaxes your eyes but also alleviates mental strain. Meet "palming," a foundational practice within the Bates Method and other vision improvement philosophies. This chapter offers a detailed examination of this age-old practice, its roots, and the tangible benefits it can bring to those looking to enhance their eyesight naturally.

The Origin of Palming

While Dr. William Bates is credited with popularizing palming in the context of vision improvement, it's essential to understand that the roots of this technique stretch far deeper. Cultures around the world have, for millennia, recognized the importance of relaxation and the powerful connection between the hands and the healing process. Indigenous and ancient healers have often placed hands over the eyes or other body parts to channel energy and promote healing.

Building on this intuitive wisdom, Bates introduced palming as a formal exercise within his method, emphasizing its role in achieving complete relaxation of both the eyes and mind.

Understanding the Technique

Palming is deceptively simple:

1. **Preparation: ** Begin by sitting comfortably at a table, ideally with a cushioned surface in front of you. Place your elbows on the table, ensuring they are well-supported.

2. **Hand Position: ** Rub your hands together briskly to generate warmth. Once warmed, place your hands over your eyes. The heel of your palms should rest on your cheekbones, with fingers on your forehead. Your palms should cup your eyes without applying pressure, ensuring no light seeps through. The fingers of one hand can overlap those of the other on the forehead.

3. **Eyes and Mind: ** Close your eyes and let them sink deep into their sockets. Imagine them floating in a dark, tranquil pool. Let go of any tension in the eye muscles. As you maintain this position, visualize calming scenes—a serene beach, a quiet forest, or any imagery that brings you peace.

4. **Duration: ** Hold this position for several minutes. Some practitioners recommend doing this for 10-15 minutes, especially when starting. Over time, you'll intuitively grasp the duration that best serves you.

The Multifaceted Benefits of Palming

- **Physical Relaxation: ** The most immediate benefit of palming is the relaxation of the eye muscles. In our screen-saturated lives, our eyes are seldom granted a break from constant stimulation. By blocking out light, palming offers the eyes a profound rest, helping alleviate strain.

- **Mental Calmness: ** The act of visualizing peaceful scenes while palming has a meditative quality. This dual focus on the eyes and the mind underscores the holistic philosophy that underpins natural vision improvement methods. As many practitioners' attest, the relaxation achieved through palming often permeates beyond the eyes, instilling a sense of overall calmness.

- **Improvement in Vision: ** Regular practitioners of palming often report a clearer and more vivid vision post the exercise. While individual experiences may vary, it's hypothesized that this clarity arises from the relaxation of the ciliary muscles and the retina's rest.

- **Alleviation of Screen Fatigue: ** In today's digital era, screen fatigue or "digital eye strain" is pervasive. Symptoms range from dry eyes to headaches and blurred vision. Integrating palming into daily routines can offer relief to those constantly tethered to screens.

A Caveat and Encouragement

Like all natural vision improvement techniques, it's essential to approach palming with an open yet discerning mind. While many swear by its benefits, it's not a magic bullet. Instead, it should be viewed as a piece of the holistic puzzle of eye care.

Moreover, the beauty of palming lies in its simplicity. It doesn't demand elaborate preparations or specialized tools. Whether you're at work taking a five-minute break or unwinding at home after a long day, palming can be seamlessly integrated into various life contexts.

In subsequent chapters, we'll delve deeper into other techniques and exercises, always with an emphasis on holistic well-being. For now, take a moment, palm your eyes, and grant yourself the gift of relaxation. Remember, the journey to perfect sight is not just about the eyes—it's about the soul too.

CHAPTER 7: SUNNING

Sunlight, the primal force of nature, has been revered across cultures and epochs as the giver of life. Beyond its ability to foster growth and sustain life, sunlight also plays a vital role in our visual health. In this chapter, we explore the practice of "sunning" — a technique leveraging controlled exposure to sunlight to benefit our eyes.

The Science Behind Sunlight and the Eyes

The human eye is an intricate organ that has evolved to function optimally in natural environments. Just as plants need sunlight for photosynthesis, our eyes require an adequate amount of natural light for proper functioning. Sunlight stimulates the production of dopamine in the eye, which can help prevent elongation of the eyeball — a key factor in myopia or short-sightedness.

Vitamin D, synthesized in our skin upon exposure to sunlight, is crucial for overall health, including the eyes. A deficiency can led to poor vision and other ocular conditions. Moreover, our eyes' natural rhythm, or the circadian cycle, is regulated by sunlight. A balance of light and darkness ensures a healthy sleep-wake pattern, which is directly linked to visual health.

Introducing the Practice of Sunning

Sunning is a controlled and deliberate exposure of the eyes to sunlight. It aims to relax the eyes, improve light adaptation, and enhance overall vision. Here's how it works:

1. **Preparation**: Find a comfortable place under direct

sunlight, preferably during the morning or late afternoon when the sun isn't at its peak. Ensure you're in a relaxed posture, either sitting or standing.

2. **Technique**: Close your eyes and face the sun directly. Feel its warmth on your eyelids. While keeping your head stationary, rotate just your eyeballs left to right, then up and down, ensuring even exposure.

3. **Duration**: Start with short intervals of 1-2 minutes, gradually increasing as you become more comfortable with the practice. Listen to your body; if it feels uncomfortable or intense, reduce the time.

4. **Post-Sunning Relaxation**: After sunning, it's beneficial to practice palming (as discussed in Chapter 6) to relax the eyes further and consolidate the benefits.

Benefits of Sunning

- **Improved Light Adaptation**: Regular sunning can enhance the eyes' ability to adapt to varying light conditions, moving from bright outdoors to dimmer indoors seamlessly.

- **Reduced Strain**: By re-acclimatizing the eyes to natural light, sunning can alleviate the strain caused by artificial lighting, especially from screens.

- **Enhanced Mood**: Exposure to sunlight increases serotonin production in the brain, promoting better mood, focus, and calmness — all of which indirectly benefit visual health.

- **Circadian Rhythm Regulation**: Maintaining a connection with the natural light-dark cycle helps regulate the body's internal clock, ensuring better sleep and overall health.

Precautions and Considerations

- **Avoid Overexposure**: Sunning should be a gentle practice. It's essential to avoid the intense midday sun, especially in hotter climates, to prevent potential damage.

- **Listen to Your Body**: If you experience discomfort, stop immediately. Sunning should be a soothing experience.

- **Complementary Practice**: While sunning offers several benefits, it isn't a cure-all. It should be integrated into a holistic vision improvement regimen, along with other practices and a balanced lifestyle.

- **Consultation**: If you have pre-existing eye conditions or concerns, it's wise to consult with an ophthalmologist or optometrist before starting sunning or any other natural vision improvement method.

In conclusion, sunning invites us to reconnect with nature, to remember that our eyes, like the rest of our body, thrive best in natural environments. As with all practices discussed in this book, the aim is holistic wellness. Embracing the sun not only illuminates our external world but also brings a little brightness into the internal landscapes of our lives. As we journey further into understanding natural vision improvement, may we always remain attuned to the simple, profound gifts that nature offers us.

CHAPTER 8: THE ROLE OF EMOTIONS AND STRESS IN VISION

For centuries, the eye has been metaphorically regarded as a window to the soul, embodying our emotional depth and the mysteries of the human psyche. While we often associate eyesight with the physiological mechanics of the eye, emerging research suggests that our emotional health can have a profound effect on our vision.

The Intricate Link Between Vision and Emotions

The relationship between vision and emotion is not merely poetic; it's deeply rooted in our physiology. Emotional stress triggers the release of adrenaline. This "fight or flight" hormone prepares our bodies for immediate action. But when this stress becomes chronic, prolonged adrenaline release can lead to visual symptoms. This can manifest as blurred vision, eye twitching, or even temporary vision loss.

Additionally, the muscles around our eyes tighten when we are stressed or anxious, which can cause strain. This is particularly prevalent in today's digital age, where screen use is omnipresent. Emotional tension, combined with the physical act of staring at screens without regular breaks, can significantly exacerbate visual stress.

Emotions and Eye Conditions

Specific emotional states have been linked to certain eye conditions:
- **Myopia (near-sightedness) **: Some studies suggest that children who are more introverted or anxious may have a higher chance of developing myopia. The reasons are multifaceted, from the physical (spending more time indoors with close-up activities) to the psychological (a desire to 'withdraw' from the outside world).

- **Central Serous Retinopathy**: This condition, where fluid builds up under the retina, has been linked to stress, type A personalities, and even sleep apnoea. Those affected often have a history of prolonged emotional stress or trauma.

- **Blepharospasm**: An uncontrollable twitch or involuntary closure of the eyelids can be exacerbated by fatigue, tension, or stress.

Techniques to Manage Emotional and Mental Stress for Better Vision

Understanding the psychological impact on vision is only the first step. Actively incorporating techniques to manage emotional and mental stress is crucial for maintaining optimal eyesight.

1. **Mindfulness and Meditation**: Engaging in mindfulness exercises and meditation can help alleviate stress. By bringing our focus to the present moment and practicing deep breathing, we can release tension in the body, including the eyes.

2. **Eye Relaxation Exercises**: Close your eyes and visualize a peaceful scene. This mental imagery, combined with palming (as discussed in Chapter 6), can provide immediate relief from visual strain.

3. **Physical Activity**: Regular physical exercise can reduce adrenaline levels and release endorphins, natural stress-

relievers. Even a short walk can help refresh the eyes and mind.

4. **Digital Detox**: Reducing screen time, especially before bed, can lessen digital eye strain and improve sleep quality.

5. **Talk Therapy**: Emotional stresses, traumas, or unresolved issues can contribute to visual problems. Speaking with a counsellor or therapist can offer coping strategies and healing.

6. **Balanced Diet**: As detailed in Chapter 20, a nutrient-rich diet can bolster eye health. Foods high in antioxidants, Vitamin A, and Omega-3 fatty acids can counteract the effects of stress on the eyes.

In conclusion, recognizing the interplay between our emotional health and vision is pivotal in our quest for perfect sight. Eyesight is not merely about the eyes' physical health but is intricately tied to our emotional well-being. By addressing and managing our emotional and mental stresses, we can journey towards achieving clearer vision without the crutch of glasses.

CHAPTER 9: IMPORTANCE OF REGULAR EYE EXERCISE'S

For many, the idea of exercising the eyes sounds perplexing. We're accustomed to the notion of exercising our bodies, strengthening our muscles, and enhancing our cardiovascular health. But when it comes to our eyes, often, we relegate their care to annual check-ups and the occasional purchase of corrective lenses. However, just as the rest of our body benefits from regular movement and challenge, our eyes thrive when given similar attention.

The "Muscle Memory" of Eyes and Why Exercise is Key

The human eye is a marvel of biology, consisting not just of the cornea, lens, and retina, but also of intricate muscles that allow it to focus, move, and adjust to different light conditions. The idea of "muscle memory" in the context of the eyes refers to the habitual patterns our eye muscles adopt over time. Whether it's the daily strain of staring at a computer screen or reading in dim lighting, these patterns can lead to the degradation of our visual acuity.

Like any muscle in the body, the muscles surrounding the eye can become stiff and unyielding if not exercised. They can lose their flexibility, making it harder to focus on objects at varying distances or adjust to changing light conditions. Regular eye exercises help maintain and restore this flexibility, potentially slowing the progression of certain visual impairments and, in some cases, even reversing them.

Simple Daily Routines to Maintain Optimal Vision

Embracing regular eye exercises can lead to noticeable improvements in vision and overall eye comfort. Here are some straightforward routines one can integrate into daily life:

1. **Blinking**: In today's screen-centric world, we tend to blink less frequently, leading to eye strain. Make a conscious effort to blink every 3-4 seconds when using digital devices. This moistens the eyes and reduces fatigue.

2. **Near and Far Focus**:
   - Sit or stand comfortably.
   - Hold your thumb about 10 inches away from your face and focus on it.
   - After a few seconds, shift your focus to an object about 10-20 feet away.
   - Alternate focus between your thumb and the distant object for a minute or two.

3. **Figure Eight**:
   - Imagine a giant figure eight on the floor about 10 feet in front of you.
   - Trace the figure eight with your eyes slowly, without moving your head.
   - Do this for a minute, then switch directions.

4. **20-20-20 Rule**: Every 20 minutes, take a 20-second break and focus on something 20 feet away. This simple rule can drastically reduce digital eye strain.

5. **Palming** (as discussed in Chapter 6):
   - Rub your hands together until they're warm.

- Close your eyes and gently place your palms over them without pressing.
- Relax and take deep breaths, visualizing darkness. Continue for 2-3 minutes.

6. **Eye Rolling**:
   - Sit up straight and look forward.
   - Look up without moving your head, then circle your eyes in a clockwise direction.
   - Take a moment, and then do the same counter clockwise. Repeat a few times.

7. **Double Thumb Technique**:
   - Extend both arms in front of you.
   - Focus on one thumb as you slowly move it closer to your nose.
   - Switch focus to the other thumb as you bring it closer. Alternate between thumbs.

8. **Visualization**: Close your eyes and visualize a place, object, or scene in great detail. This practice not only relaxes the mind but also gives the eyes a much-needed break.

The key to these exercises is consistency. Much like physical workouts, the benefits accrue over time. They work best when they're a part of a daily routine, ensuring your eyes remain flexible, healthy, and sharp.

In conclusion, the significance of regular eye exercises cannot be overstated. Just as our bodies need movement to stay agile and fit, our eyes require consistent stimulation and challenge. Integrating these simple routines into daily life can lead to improved vision, reduced eye strain, and a greater sense of well-being. After all, our eyes are not just windows to the world; they're windows to our soul's perception of that world.

CHAPTER 10: BLINKING AND ITS BENEFITS

Blinking, a seemingly insignificant and reflexive action, plays a pivotal role in maintaining and even improving our vision. Blinking is as fundamental to eye health as breathing is to life. While often taken for granted, this simple act holds profound benefits that, when harnessed consciously, can offer significant improvements to our visual well-being.

The Science Behind Blinking

Blinking serves several essential purposes for our eyes:

1. **Lubrication**: Each time we blink, a thin layer of tears spreads across the cornea, the eye's outermost surface. This tear film serves multiple roles: it keeps the eye moist, offers essential nutrients, and removes micro-debris that might enter the eye.

2. **Protection**: Blinking acts as a natural defence mechanism against potential irritants like dust, smoke, and other airborne particles. The eyelids' swift motion during a blink can help dislodge and flush out these particles.

3. **Nutrient Distribution**: The tears produced during blinking are not merely water. They contain a mix of oils, mucus, antibodies, and over 1500 different proteins essential for eye health. Blinking ensures a fresh supply of these nutrients every few seconds.

4. **Vision Clarity**: A continuous tear film is pivotal for maintaining clear vision. It refracts light entering the eye, ensuring that it's focused precisely on the retina. Disruptions to this tear film, often caused by reduced blinking, can lead to vision distortions.

Why Regular and Conscious Blinking Can Improve Vision

In our modern world dominated by screens, the frequency and quality of our blinks have been affected. Staring at computer monitors, smartphones, or televisions can reduce our blink rate by nearly half, leading to digital eye strain or "computer vision syndrome." This syndrome can manifest as dry eyes, blurred vision, and even headaches. Here's where conscious blinking comes into play.

1. **Counteracting Dry Eyes**: Regular and full blinks can combat the sensation of dry eyes. A complete blink — where the upper eyelid touches the lower eyelid — ensures that the tear film is evenly spread across the cornea. Partial blinks, common during screen time, can leave the lower part of the cornea uncovered, leading to dryness.

2. **Reducing Eye Strain**: Blinking offers the eye muscles a brief respite. Given that we blink about 15 times a minute, this translates to a 10% reduction in visual information the brain needs to process. This small break can significantly reduce the strain on our eye muscles and the brain, especially during prolonged periods of focus.

3. **Enhancing Focus**: Regular blinking can actually sharpen our focus. With each blink, the eye undergoes a momentary period of darkness which can help in resetting our visual system, allowing us to focus better on the subsequent visual information.

4. **Removing Toxins**: Blinking activates the eye's drainage system, the puncta, which flushes the tears into the nose. This

drainage not only carries away physical debris but also various toxins that might have accumulated in the tear film.

5. **Promoting Relaxation**: Much like deep breaths in meditation, conscious blinking can be a form of relaxation. Pausing to take a few deliberate blinks can calm the mind and reduce overall stress, which in turn benefits our eyes.

To reap the full benefits of blinking, one must practice it consciously, especially during activities that reduce our natural blink reflex. Simple techniques include:

- **20-20-20 Rule**: Every 20 minutes, take a 20-second break, and blink consciously 20 times.

- **Full Blinking**: Practice full and deliberate blinks, ensuring the upper eyelid meets the lower eyelid with each blink.

- **Mindful Breaks**: Periodically detach from screens or intensive tasks and take a minute to just blink and look around, allowing the eyes to reset.

In conclusion, while blinking might appear inconsequential, it's a powerhouse of benefits for our eyes. It reminds us of nature's wisdom — how something so simple, so reflexive, holds the key to our visual well-being. By recognizing its importance and practicing conscious blinking, we can not only protect our eyes but significantly enhance our vision and overall eye health.

CHAPTER 11: CENTRAL FIXATION PRINCIPLE

In our journey to understand vision holistically, we arrive at a crucial juncture — the principle of central fixation. This principle, although not widely discussed in contemporary eye care, holds significant value for those aiming for natural vision improvement. Central fixation emphasizes the idea that we see best at the point where we're looking directly. In essence, it's about harnessing the full potential of our eyes' focal point. Let's delve deeper into this concept.

The Concept of Seeing Best Where You're Looking Directly

1. **The Anatomy Behind Central Fixation**: The retina, located at the back of our eyes, contains millions of light-sensitive cells. However, not all parts of the retina are created equal. The centre, called the macula, and more specifically, its innermost part, the fovea, contains the highest concentration of cone cells, responsible for our central and colour vision. When we look directly at something, the image falls on the fovea. Given its rich cellular density, the fovea is the point of sharpest vision.

2. **Peripheral vs. Central Vision**: While our eyes are designed to provide a broad visual field, not everything within this field is seen with the same clarity. Objects directly in our line of sight (central vision) are perceived with utmost precision, whereas those in the periphery are seen less distinctly. Central fixation

is about maximizing this disparity to our advantage — training our eyes and brain to focus on what's directly ahead and letting the rest fade into the background.

3. **The Mental Component**: Central fixation isn't just about the eyes; it's also about the mind. When we focus intently on one point, our brain gives it precedence over peripheral information. This mental "tunnel vision" complements our eyes' natural ability, further enhancing clarity.

Practical Exercises to Improve Central Vision

Enhancing our central vision requires practice, patience, and a bit of know-how. Here are exercises designed to tap into the power of the central fixation principle:

1. **The Dot Exercise**:
   - Find a piece of paper with printed text and identify a full stop or a comma.
   - Focus on the punctuation mark, trying to see it as clearly as possible.
   - Gradually shift your focus to the letters around it, noticing the disparity in clarity.
   - Return your focus to the punctuation, training your eyes and brain to centralize attention.

2. **The Wand Technique**:
   - Hold a pencil or a wand vertically, with its tip aligned with your eyes.
   - Focus on the tip as you slowly move the wand left and right, keeping the tip as the central point of your vision.
   - As you do this, be aware of the background moving in the opposite direction but keep your focus strictly on the wand's tip.

3. **Reading with Awareness**:
   - Choose a book or a magazine.
   - As you read, be hyper-aware of where your eyes are focusing. Your aim is to focus on one word at a time, letting the

surrounding words blur slightly.
   - With time, you'll notice your reading speed might slow down initially but will pick up with enhanced clarity as you practice.

4. **The "20-20-20" Drill with a Twist**:
   - As mentioned in the blinking chapter, every 20 minutes, take a 20-second break from screens.
   - During this break, pick an object 20 feet away and focus on its smallest detail, training your eyes to centralize vision.

5. **Mental Imagery**:
   - Close your eyes and imagine a bullseye target.
   - Focus on the centremost circle, visualizing it with utmost clarity, while letting the outer rings fade.
   - Gradually shift your mental focus to the outer rings and then back to the centre, practicing the principle of central fixation mentally.

In conclusion, the central fixation principle is a testament to the intricacy of our visual system. It reminds us that the eyes, paired with the brain, have evolved with a remarkable ability to prioritize and focus. By understanding and applying this principle through exercises, we can harness our vision's full potential, inching closer to the promise of perfect sight without glasses.

CHAPTER 12: SHIFTING AND SWINGING TECHNIQUES

In the labyrinth of vision care, the techniques of shifting and swinging stand as pillars of natural eyesight improvement. Both, at their core, are designed to bring about relaxation, improve focus, and reduce the stress our eyes endure daily, particularly in this digital age. By mastering these techniques, one not only enhances their vision but also ensures a more harmonious relationship between the eyes and the brain. Let's venture into these techniques, understanding their essence and the ways to incorporate them into our daily routines.

The Art of Moving the Eyes to Improve Focus and Reduce Strain

1. **Understanding the Need**: Contrary to common belief, our eyes are not meant to remain static. They're designed to move, to dance across what they observe, continuously adjusting and refocusing. In modern life, however, we often fixate on screens or texts, limiting our eyes' natural movement. This restriction can lead to strain and blur. Shifting and swinging are techniques that reintroduce this fluidity into our visual routine.

2. **Shifting - The Gentle Glide**: Shifting is the simple act of

moving our eyes from one point to another. It sounds basic, but doing so consciously can have profound effects. When we shift our gaze, we stimulate different parts of the retina, allowing for a brief moment of relaxation in between. It's akin to giving our eyes a mini break.

3. **Swinging - The Visual Waltz**: Swinging involves moving our entire head and allowing our eyes to follow the motion passively. The idea is to introduce a sense of motion into our visual field, promoting relaxation. Imagine standing in front of a pendulum—rather than tracking it with just our eyes, we would move our whole head to follow its swing, letting the world move before our eyes.

Guided Exercises to Practice the Shifting and Swinging

To make these techniques a part of our daily lives, practical exercises are paramount. Here are some guided steps:

1. **Shifting Exercise - The "A to B" Focus**:
   - Choose two objects or points in your vicinity.
   - Look at point A, observe its details, and then slowly shift your gaze to point B.
   - Do this back and forth for a minute, ensuring smooth transitions and not darting quickly.

2. **Shifting Exercise - "Near and Far"**:
   - Hold a finger or a pen close to your face.
   - Focus on it for a few seconds, then shift your gaze to an object farther away.
   - This exercise helps improve accommodation, the eye's ability to change its focus between near and distant objects.

3. **Swinging Exercise - The "Door Frame Technique"**:
   - Stand in a doorway, facing the frame.
   - Turn your body and head to the left, then to the right, allowing your eyes to passively observe the movement of the door frame.

- Your vision should feel fluid, with objects flowing across your visual field. The aim isn't to focus on specifics but to appreciate the motion.

4. **Swinging Exercise - "The Horizon Swing"**:
   - Stand or sit by a window, or better yet outside.
   - Focus on the horizon and slowly turn your head from left to right, letting the vastness in front of you swing across your field of view.
   - This exercise not only benefits the eyes but is also a wonderful meditative experience.

5. **Combined Exercise - "Shift-Swing Dance"**:
   - Choose a line of text in a book or on your screen.
   - Start at the beginning, shifting from word to word.
   - Once you reach the end, swing your head (and thus your gaze) to the start again.
   - This exercise is particularly beneficial for those who read or work on screens for prolonged periods.

To encapsulate, the principles of shifting and swinging are not just exercises; they are a philosophy. They teach us the importance of motion, of not letting our eyes stagnate, and of appreciating the dynamic world around us. By incorporating these techniques into our daily routine, we step closer to a life of clearer vision and reduced ocular stress, navigating our way towards perfect sight without glasses.

CHAPTER 13: DISTANCE VISION AND THE HORIZON GAZING TECHNIQUE

In a world dominated by screens, it's ironic how often we limit our vision to just a few feet in front of us. Our smartphones, tablets, computers, and televisions become the boundaries of our visual world. However, our eyes are not designed for such restrictions; they crave depth, breadth, and the infinity of the horizon. Harnessing the power of distance vision can be a significant step towards improving our eyesight, especially for those grappling with near-sightedness.

Understanding the Importance of Regularly Using Our Distance Vision

1. **Eyes Crave Variation**: Just as our minds benefit from different forms of stimulation - from intense concentration to daydreaming - our eyes too need variety. They are designed to focus both on the minuscule details of a leaf and the expansive grandeur of a mountain range. Switching between near and far focus keeps our eye muscles agile and responsive.

2. **Modern Lifestyle Challenges**: Today, especially in urban environments, our sight is often boxed in. Walls, buildings, and screens restrict the vistas our ancestors naturally enjoyed.

This limitation can lead our eyes to adapt to a predominantly near-focused state, sometimes contributing to myopia (near-sightedness).

3. **Natural Calibration**: Looking into the distance, beyond artificial lights and pixels, allows our eyes to recalibrate. The vastness, natural light, and varied depth perception can serve as a kind of 'reset' for our vision, aligning it to its natural state.

How Gazing into the Distance Can Help with Near-sightedness

1. **Reversing the Strain**: One of the theories behind the development of myopia is the consistent strain placed on the eyes due to close-up work, be it reading, writing, or screen time. By consciously spending time gazing at distant objects, we can counterbalance this strain, giving the eyes a chance to relax and the eye muscles an opportunity to stretch.

2. **Stimulating the Peripheral Vision**: Distant gazing, especially at expansive views like horizons, stimulates not just the central but also the peripheral vision. This holistic visual engagement is both relaxing and invigorating for the eyes.

3. **Horizon Gazing Technique – A Guided Approach**:

   - **Choosing the Right Spot**: Start by finding a location that offers an expansive view. It could be a park, a beach, a hilltop, or even a tall building in the city that overlooks a vast landscape.

   - **Positioning**: Stand or sit comfortably. Ensure that you're in a relaxed posture. Take a few deep breaths to centre yourself.

   - **Soft Gaze**: Instead of trying to focus intently on one object, let your gaze be soft and expansive. Absorb the vastness in front of you. Feel the depth and the breadth of the view.

   - **Time**: Spend at least 10 minutes in this activity. However, the longer you can practice horizon gazing, the better. Over time, try to integrate this into your daily routine, even if it's just looking out of a window for a few minutes every hour.

- **Mindfulness**: While this is an exercise for the eyes, it can also be a meditative experience. As you gaze out, be present. Let go of other thoughts and immerse yourself in the moment and the view.

- **Frequency**: Aim to practice horizon gazing daily, especially if you spend significant hours working up close or on screens. Think of it as a kind of visual meditation, a break for both your eyes and your mind.

In conclusion, the act of looking into the distance is not just about what lies yonder; it's a journey inward, to the innate abilities of our eyes. The horizon gazing technique isn't just an exercise; it's a return to our natural state, a reminder of the boundless vistas our eyes are meant to explore. Embracing distance vision can be a pivotal step in our journey toward perfect sight without glasses. After all, in gazing at the horizon, we're not just seeing the world; we're also understanding a bit more about ourselves.

CHAPTER 14: PRINT PUSHING FOR NEAR-SIGHTEDNESS

Print pushing is a term that might initially seem paradoxical. Given the rampant concerns regarding screen time and excessive reading as potential culprits for vision problems, it's counterintuitive to think of reading as a remedy. Yet, when done correctly, "print pushing" can be a valuable method to alleviate the symptoms of myopia, or near-sightedness. Let's delve deeper into this technique, understand its underlying principles, and learn how to harness its potential for improving vision.

A Method to Gradually Improve Myopia by Reading

1. **Understanding Myopia**: Before diving into the technique, it's essential to have a brief overview of myopia. People with myopia can see close objects clearly, but distant objects appear blurred. This blurring is due to the elongation of the eye, causing light rays to focus in front of the retina rather than directly on it.

2. **Print Pushing Defined**: Print pushing involves reading text from a distance where it's just barely clear and gradually increasing that distance as your eyes adjust. The goal is to challenge the eyes slightly, prompting them to adapt, but without causing undue strain.

3. **The Science Behind Print Pushing**: The idea is to reduce the "hyperopic defocus." In simpler terms, when someone with

myopia focuses on near objects, the image forms behind the retina. By pushing the print further away, we aim to reduce this defocus, guiding the eye to correct its elongation over time and bring the image formation back onto the retina.

Guidelines on How to Effectively Use the Print Pushing Technique

1. **Starting Point**: Begin with a book or any printed material. The print should be of standard size, not too large or too small. Find a spot where the text is clear but right at the edge of clarity. This is your starting point.

2. **Gradual Movement**: As you read, slowly push the material away from you until the print starts to blur slightly. The aim is not to strain your eyes but to challenge them. If you find yourself squinting or feeling any discomfort, you've pushed too far.

3. **Consistency is Key**: Like any exercise, consistency yields result. Dedicate a specific time daily, perhaps 20-30 minutes, solely for print pushing. Over time, you should find that you can start your reading session from a farther distance than you initially could.

4. **Proper Lighting**: Ensure that you're reading in good light. Dim light can cause you to strain, which is counterproductive to the print pushing technique.

5. **Maintain Good Posture**: Sit in a comfortable position, keeping your back straight. Your reading material should be at eye level, ensuring that you aren't looking down or up at a steep angle.

6. **Document Your Progress**: Keep a journal to note the distance you start at and the distance you reach by the end of your session. Tracking your progress can be motivating and will give you tangible evidence of improvement.

7. **Rest and Blink**: Don't forget to blink regularly as you read.

If you feel any fatigue, close your eyes for a few moments, take a deep breath, and then continue.

8. **Supplement with Other Techniques**: While print pushing can be effective, it's beneficial when combined with other natural vision improvement methods, such as sunning, palming, or the Bates method.

9. **Avoid Close Tasks After a Session**: After a print pushing session, try to avoid very close tasks like smartphone scrolling or detailed artwork. Give your eyes some time to adapt and rest.

10. **Consultation**: If you're starting with a high degree of myopia, it's beneficial to consult with an optometrist familiar with natural vision improvement techniques. They can guide you more effectively based on your individual needs.

In conclusion, print pushing is a testament to the adaptability of the human body, specifically our eyes. While it might seem like a simple technique, its foundations lie in the intricate dance of muscles, lenses, and light. By challenging our eyes in a measured manner, we not only aim to improve our vision but also reconnect with the inherent capabilities they possess. With dedication, patience, and consistent practice, many have found print pushing to be a beacon on their journey to perfect sight without glasses.

CHAPTER 15: THE SNELLEN CHART: MORE THAN JUST AN EYE TEST

Most of us, at some point in our lives, have found ourselves seated in an optometrist's office, staring at a chart with progressively smaller letters, trying our best to decipher those elusive lines as they blur into obscurity. That chart, known as the Snellen Chart, is a staple in ophthalmology clinics worldwide. But did you know that apart from its diagnostic use, the Snellen Chart can also serve as a tool for vision improvement?

History and Purpose of the Snellen Chart

1. **Origins of the Chart**: The Snellen Chart traces its origins to the 1860s when a Dutch ophthalmologist named Herman Snellen designed it. Snellen aimed to create a standardized way to measure visual acuity. Before this, there wasn't a consistent method, making it challenging to compare and contrast results or diagnose vision conditions accurately.

2. **Understanding "20/20" Vision**: One term frequently associated with the Snellen Chart is "20/20 vision." This means that a person can see clearly at 20 feet what should normally be seen at that distance. If someone has 20/40 vision, it implies

they must be at 20 feet to see what a person with 20/20 vision can see at 40 feet.

3. **Design and Logic**: The chart typically consists of eleven lines of block letters. Each line represents a certain level of visual acuity. As the lines descend, the letters become smaller, challenging the eyes more. The design ensures a precise measurement of how well one can discern details and contrast at a standardized distance.

Using the Snellen Chart as a Daily Vision Exercise

While the primary function of the Snellen Chart is diagnostic, it can also serve as a tool for vision improvement when used intentionally and consciously. Here's how:

1. **Familiarization**: Start by understanding the chart. Print a standard Snellen Chart and hang it in a well-lit room at eye level. Ensure you can stand or sit 20 feet away from it, emulating the conditions you'd find in an optometrist's office.

2. **Daily Reading**: Spend a few minutes each day reading the chart, starting from the top and working your way down to the smallest line you can read without straining. The aim is not to stress your eyes but to challenge them gently.

3. **Blinking and Relaxation**: As you read the chart, remember to blink frequently. Blinking moistens the eyes and provides brief moments of relaxation, crucial for maintaining eye health. If a particular line feels challenging, close your eyes, take a few deep breaths, and try again.

4. **Active Focus**: Instead of passively reading the letters, actively engage with them. Observe the spaces between the letters, the contours of each letter, and the contrast between the letters and the background. This active engagement can enhance your central fixation and help improve your focus over time.

5. **Chart Variations**: To further challenge your eyes, consider using variations of the Snellen Chart. Some versions use tumbling E's or Landolt rings instead of letters. Switching between different charts can present novel challenges to your eyes, promoting adaptability and flexibility.

6. **Progress Tracking**: Just as with the print pushing technique, it can be motivating to track your progress. Note the smallest line you can read comfortably each day. Over time, with consistent practice, you might notice improvements in your visual acuity.

7. **Pair with Other Techniques**: While the Snellen Chart exercise is beneficial on its own, it's even more effective when paired with other vision improvement methods. Consider combining your daily Snellen reading with techniques like palming, sunning, or swinging for a comprehensive vision workout.

8. **Consultation**: As always, if you're starting with a pronounced vision problem or if you're unsure about any aspect of the exercise, consult an optometrist familiar with natural vision improvement techniques.

In essence, the Snellen Chart, often seen as a mere diagnostic tool, holds untapped potential for those keen on natural vision improvement. With conscious effort, this age-old chart can be repurposed from a mere tester of eyesight into a trainer, guiding us closer to the goal of perfect sight without glasses.

CHAPTER 16: COLOUR THERAPY AND VISION

The Impact of Different Colours on Our Eyes and Mood

Colours are more than just visual stimulants; they have profound psychological and physiological impacts on our minds and bodies. From the tranquillity evoked by a soft blue to the warmth of a fiery red, colours influence our moods, feelings, and even our physical wellbeing. This influence extends to our eyes and how we perceive the world.

Blue, for instance, is often associated with calmness, serenity, and relaxation. It is the colour of clear skies and deep oceans, evoking feelings of spaciousness and peace. On the eyes, blue light, especially from screens, can be straining if overly exposed. However, naturally occurring blue tones, like those of the sky at dawn or dusk, can be restful and help reduce eye fatigue.

Red, a colour of passion, urgency, and alertness, can stimulate the mind and body. It can also increase heart rate and raise blood pressure. For the eyes, looking at red can be energizing, but overexposure might be overstimulating, causing discomfort.

Green, the colour of nature, is balanced and calming. It can reduce anxiety and is known to relieve stress. For our eyes, green, especially the shade seen in natural environments like forests, can be soothing and can help alleviate eye strain.

Yellow, the colour of sunshine, is uplifting and can stimulate mental processes and the nervous system. When it comes to our eyes, yellow can be bright and may cause some discomfort if it's too intense. However, softer yellow tones can be comforting.

How to Use Colour Therapy for Vision Improvement

Harnessing the power of colours for better vision involves mindful practices and intentional incorporation of colours into our environment. Here are some steps and techniques:

1. **Natural Environment**: Spend time in nature. Green, being a dominant colour in many natural landscapes, helps in reducing eye strain. Nature walks can not only improve vision but also provide psychological benefits.

2. **Limit Blue Light Exposure**: While blue has calming effects in natural settings, blue light from digital devices can strain the eyes. Limit screen time, especially before bedtime, and consider using blue light filters on your devices.

3. **Coloured Filters for Reading**: Some people find that using coloured overlays or filters when reading can reduce strain and improve clarity. The ideal colour varies from person to person, so experimenting with different hues can help determine the best one for you.

4. **Meditation with Colours**: Close your eyes and visualize calming colours. This not only relaxes the mind but also gives the eyes a break from constant visual stimulation. Alternatively, meditating in a room with coloured light bulbs can create a calming ambiance that benefits both mood and eyesight.

5. **Balanced Light Sources**: Ensure that you're living and working spaces are well-lit but avoid overly harsh lighting. Soft white or yellow light can be easier on the eyes than stark white or cool blue lights.

6. **Wear the Right Shades**: Sunglasses aren't just a fashion statement; they protect the eyes from harmful UV rays and intense light. opt for polarized lenses that reduce glare and

choose tints that are comfortable for your eyes.

7. **Diversify Your Palette**: Surround yourself with a variety of colours. This allows your eyes to adjust to different shades, intensities, and contrasts, which can be a form of exercise for them.

8. **Seek Professional Guidance**: If you're keen on exploring colour therapy in-depth, consider consulting a therapist specializing in this area. They can provide tailored advice and techniques based on your individual needs.

In conclusion, while colour therapy is not a replacement for professional medical advice and practices, it offers supplementary benefits. By understanding the effects of different colours on our eyes and moods, we can create an environment that promotes both mental and visual well-being. Remember, our eyes, like every other part of our body, need care, rest, and a balanced environment to function optimally.

CHAPTER 17: THE MEMORY AND IMAGINATION CONNECTION

How Visualization Exercises Can Aid in Vision Correction

The connection between the mind and the body is profound, and the eyes are no exception to this interplay. Our eyes not only perceive the world but are also influenced by our internal states, including memory and imagination. Visualization exercises tap into these faculties to support vision correction.

One reason visualization can be influential is due to the brain's plasticity. Just as muscles can be trained and strengthened, neural pathways in the brain can be moulded and adapted through practice. Visualization exercises leverage this adaptability to foster positive changes in the eyes.

When we visualize, we stimulate the same neural circuits as when we're physically seeing. Engaging the visual centers of the brain through memory and imagination exercises can help reinforce and even rebuild weakened visual pathways, aiding in vision correction.

Techniques to Harness the Power of Memory and Imagination for Better Sight

1. **Palming Visualization**:
   - Start by palming: Rub your hands together to create warmth, then gently cup your eyes without pressing the eyelids.
   - In this relaxed state, recall a pleasant memory with vivid visual details. Relive the colours, shapes, and spatial dimensions. Feel the joy of that memory seep into your eyes through the warmth of your palms. This exercise combines relaxation with positive visual stimulation.

2. **Dynamic Visualization**:
   - Close your eyes and imagine a pendulum swinging from left to right. Follow the pendulum in your mind's eye as it moves, ensuring that your eyeballs don't move.
   - Gradually make the pendulum move faster or incorporate more complex patterns. This exercise trains the brain to keep up with dynamic visual information and strengthens eye muscles without physical movement.

3. **Positive Reinforcement through Memory**:
   - Recall a moment when your vision was sharp and clear. Relive the satisfaction and clarity of that moment.
   - Now, anchor that feeling. Whenever you experience moments of clear vision, consciously acknowledge and store that feeling. Over time, your brain will associate this positive reinforcement with clear vision, promoting better sight.

4. **Visualization of Text**:
   - Remember a passage from a book, an article, or a signboard you recently read. Visualize the text in your mind as clearly as possible.
   - Imagine the font type, size, and the background colour. Then try to read the text in your mind's eye. This exercise enhances your brain's ability to process textual information, beneficial for those who have reading-related vision problems.

5. **Distance Visualization**:
   - Picture a distant scene, such as a horizon, a mountain range,

or a skyline. Visualize the far-off details and colours.

- Over time, challenge yourself by adding more intricate details. This exercise helps individuals with myopia (short-sightedness) train their brains to process distant visuals.

6. **Face Recall**:
   - Think of a loved one or a famous personality. Remember their facial features in detail – the eyes, nose, lips, and expressions.
   - This exercise aids in enhancing focus and facial recognition abilities, which can sometimes be problematic for those with vision impairments.

7. **Guided Imagery Sessions**:
   - Listening to guided imagery audio can be beneficial. The narrator describes a scene, and you visualize it, allowing your brain to construct images based on verbal cues. This practice can enhance the connection between auditory and visual centers, promoting better vision.

8. **Meditative Visualization**:
   - In a meditative state, visualize a healing light encompassing your eyes. Imagine this light penetrating and healing any imperfections.
   - Though this technique is more metaphysical than the others, many find solace and reported improvements in vision with regular practice.

In essence, the brain's ability to remember and imagine is a powerful tool in the quest for natural vision improvement. Like any other form of training, consistency is key. Regularly practicing these exercises can create a significant impact over time. Remember that while these techniques are valuable, they should complement, not replace, professional medical advice and treatments.

CHAPTER 18: THE ROLE OF SLEEP AND REST IN VISION HEALTH

The Science of How Eyes Rejuvenate During Sleep

Sleep is a fundamental requirement for overall health, and its significance in vision health cannot be overstated. During sleep, our body goes into a mode of recovery and rejuvenation. This restorative process is particularly crucial for our eyes, which are in constant use when we are awake.

1. **Cellular Repair**: Every day, due to exposure to light, environmental pollutants, and regular wear and tear, the cells of our eyes experience damage. During the deeper stages of sleep, the repair of these cells takes place. This ensures that the delicate structures, particularly the retina and cornea, are restored and prepared for the next day.

2. **Nutrient Replenishment**: The eyes, especially the retina, have a high metabolic rate. During waking hours, these cells consume nutrients to function. Sleep allows the metabolic processes to balance out, replenishing the consumed nutrients and removing waste products.

3. **Reduction of Eye Fatigue**: Just like our muscles get tired after prolonged use, the muscles in our eyes can also get

fatigued, leading to blurred vision or even strain. Sleep gives these muscles the necessary break to recover.

4. **Lubrication Restoration**: Blinking spreads tear film over the eyes, ensuring they remain moist. While awake, environmental factors and prolonged screen time can dry the eyes. Sleep provides an extended period for the eyes to maintain a consistent tear film, restoring optimal lubrication.

5. **Clearing Out Debris**: Throughout the day, tiny debris and particles can get into our eyes. The glymphatic system, which clears waste from the brain and eyes, is more active during sleep. This system helps in flushing out potential harmful debris from the eyes.

Tips for a Restful Sleep for Optimal Vision

1. **Establish a Routine**: Going to bed and waking up at the same time daily, even on weekends, helps regulate the body's internal clock and improves the quality of sleep.

2. **Create a Sleep-friendly Environment**: Ensure your bedroom is dark, quiet, and cool. Consider using blackout curtains, earplugs, or white noise machines if necessary.

3. **Limit Screen Time Before Bed**: The blue light emitted by screens can interfere with the production of melatonin, the hormone responsible for sleep. Try to avoid screens at least an hour before bedtime.

4. **Mind Your Diet**: Avoid caffeine or heavy meals close to bedtime. They can disrupt sleep. Instead, opt for sleep-inducing foods like almonds, chamomile tea, or warm milk.

5. **Engage in Relaxation Techniques**: Incorporate practices such as reading, meditating, or deep-breathing exercises before bed. These can help calm the mind and prepare the body for restful sleep.

6. **Optimize Your Sleep Position**: Sleeping face down can put

pressure on the eyes. Try sleeping on your back or side to minimize any unnecessary pressure.

7. **Stay Hydrated**: Proper hydration supports tear production. Ensure you drink adequate water throughout the day, but limit intake right before sleep to avoid midnight trips to the bathroom.

8. **Reduce Alcohol and Tobacco Consumption**: Both can interfere with sleep patterns. Limiting or avoiding their consumption, especially closer to bedtime, can lead to better sleep quality.

9. **Evaluate Your Bedding**: A good mattress and pillow can significantly improve sleep quality. Make sure they provide adequate support and are comfortable.

10. **Consult a Sleep Specialist**: If you have trouble sleeping or feel constantly tired during the day, it might be a good idea to see a sleep specialist. Conditions like sleep apnoea can have profound effects on overall health, including vision.

In conclusion, sleep is not merely a time of rest for the body and mind, but it's a crucial period of restoration and rejuvenation for the eyes. The link between sleep and vision health is undeniable, and by ensuring we get quality sleep, we take a significant step towards maintaining clear and healthy vision. Just as we prioritize other aspects of eye care, prioritizing sleep is equally essential for optimal eye health.

CHAPTER 19: UNDERSTANDING AND COMBATING EYE FATIGUE

Causes and Symptoms of Eye Strain

Eye fatigue, often referred to as eye strain or asthenopia, is a common condition that arises when the eyes get tired from prolonged use, such as staring at a screen or driving long distances. Understanding the causes and recognizing the symptoms is the first step in addressing and alleviating the issue.

*Causes of Eye Fatigue: *

1. **Prolonged Screen Time**: In our digital age, one of the primary causes is extended periods spent looking at screens. Computers, smartphones, tablets, and televisions emit blue light, which can be particularly straining for the eyes.

2. **Improper Lighting**: Working in too dim or too bright lighting conditions can put additional stress on the eyes.

3. **Extended Focus on Close-Up Tasks**: Activities like reading, writing, or handcrafting for long durations without breaks can lead to eye fatigue.

4. **Driving for Long Periods**: Constant focus on the road,

especially in challenging conditions like rain or night-time, can strain the eyes.

5. **Incorrect Prescription**: Wearing glasses or contact lenses with outdated or incorrect prescriptions can force the eyes to work harder, leading to fatigue.

6. **Underlying Eye Conditions**: Dry eye, uncorrected vision problems, or slight misalignment of the eyes can contribute to quicker onset of eye fatigue.

*Symptoms of Eye Fatigue: *

- Sore or irritated eyes
- Dry or watery eyes
- Blurred or double vision
- Increased sensitivity to light
- Difficulty concentrating
- Headaches
- Pain in the neck, shoulders, or back

Best Practices to Avoid and Alleviate Eye Fatigue

1. **Follow the 20-20-20 Rule**: Every 20 minutes, take a 20-second break and focus on something at least 20 feet away. This simple practice allows your eye muscles to relax.

2. **Adjust Lighting**: Ensure that your workspace has proper lighting. Avoid glare on screens from windows or lights. Using an anti-glare screen protector can also be beneficial.

3. **Blink Regularly**: Blinking moistens the eyes, reducing dryness and discomfort. When focused, especially on screens, we tend to blink less, so make a conscious effort to blink more often.

4. **Optimize Screen Settings**: Increase text size for comfortable reading. Adjust the contrast and brightness levels to be in sync with your surroundings. Consider using blue light filters, especially in the evenings.

5. **Correct Your Posture**: Ensure you're sitting at a comfortable height with the screen at eye level or slightly below. Your feet should be flat on the ground, and your back should be supported.

6. **Keep the Screen at a Distance**: Ideally, the screen should be about an arm's length away. Adjust the distance to where you can comfortably read the text without leaning forward.

7. **Regular Eye Examinations**: Regular check-ups will ensure that any underlying vision problems are detected and addressed, reducing the chances of eye fatigue.

8. **Stay Hydrated**: Drink plenty of water throughout the day. Hydration supports eye moisture, reducing symptoms of dryness.

9. **Use Artificial Tears**: Over-the-counter lubricating eye drops can help in relieving dryness and discomfort.

10. **Practice Palming**: Rub your hands together to generate heat, then gently cup your eyes without pressing. The warmth and darkness provide a refreshing break for the eyes.

11. **Modify Your Environment**: Use humidifiers if the air in your environment is dry. Positioning your desk so that windows are to the side, rather than in front or behind, can also minimize glare.

12. **Eye Exercises**: Simple exercises, like rolling your eyes or focusing on a close object and then a distant one repeatedly, can help reduce strain.

13. **Ensure Proper Sleep**: Adequate rest is essential. Ensure you're getting enough sleep to allow your eyes to recover from the day's exertions.

In conclusion, our eyes, like any other part of our body, can get tired and need adequate care and breaks. By recognizing the signs of fatigue and implementing the best practices outlined above, we can protect our eyes and ensure they function optimally. In the long run, consistent care can not only alleviate immediate discomfort but also contribute to better overall vision health.

Part III: Lifestyle and Eyesight

CHAPTER 20: DIET AND VISION

The saying, "You are what you eat," resonates profoundly when discussing vision and ocular health. Diet plays a paramount role in our overall health and well-being, and its effects on vision are unequivocal. Just as a well-oiled machine function flawlessly, providing our eyes with the right nutrients ensures they work optimally and remain healthy. This chapter delves deep into the connection between diet and vision, highlighting the essential nutrients that can significantly influence eye health.

The Nutrient-Eye Connection

Our eyes, much like other organs, rely on specific nutrients to function efficiently. The lack of these nutrients can not only hinder performance but also predispose the eye to several disorders. On the other hand, a diet rich in particular vitamins and minerals can enhance visual clarity, delay the onset of age-related issues, and fortify the eyes against potential diseases.

Essential Nutrients for Eye Health

1. **Vitamin A**: Known as the "vision vitamin," Vitamin A is crucial for maintaining good vision, especially in low-light conditions. A deficiency can led to conditions such as night blindness. It also plays a role in maintaining a clear cornea, the outside covering of your eye.
   - *Sources*: Carrots, sweet potatoes, spinach, and kale.

2. **Vitamin C**: This antioxidant helps protect the eyes against

damaging UV rays by absorbing more of these rays. It's considered helpful in preventing or delaying cataracts and age-related macular degeneration.
   - *Sources*: Citrus fruits like oranges and grapefruits, strawberries, bell peppers, and broccoli.

3. **Vitamin E**: Another potent antioxidant, Vitamin E guards against oxidative damage that can lead to macular degeneration and cataracts.
   - *Sources*: Nuts, seeds, and green leafy vegetables.

4. **Zinc**: This mineral plays a vital role in bringing vitamin A from the liver to the retina to produce melanin, a protective pigment in the eyes.
   - *Sources*: Beef, poultry, oysters, cereals, and dairy products.

5. **Omega-3 Fatty Acids**: These are essential fats our body can't produce. They play a crucial role in visual development and retinal function. Omega-3s can also help prevent dry eyes.
   - *Sources*: Fish like salmon, flaxseeds, and walnuts.

6. **Lutein and Zeaxanthin**: These are carotenoids found in the retina, and they protect the eyes from harmful high-energy light waves like ultraviolet rays.
   - *Sources*: Spinach, kale, peas, and eggs.

7. **Beta Carotene**: When combined with zinc and vitamins C and E, beta carotene may reduce the progression of macular degeneration.
   - *Sources*: Carrots, sweet potatoes, spinach, and kale.

8. **Bioflavonoids**: They may protect against cataracts and macular degeneration.
   - *Sources*: Citrus fruits, berries, onions, tea, and red wine.

Holistic Approach to Diet and Vision

While focusing on these nutrients is vital, it's equally essential to remember the bigger picture: overall dietary habits and patterns play a critical role. A balanced diet, rich in colorful fruits and vegetables, provides not just these nutrients but also countless other beneficial compounds that promote general and ocular health.

Moreover, some habits can be detrimental to visual health. Excessive sugar intake, for example, can increase the risk of diabetic retinopathy, while high sodium intake might elevate the risk of cataracts. A diet high in saturated fats can also pose risks. Therefore, moderation is key.

In Conclusion

Dietary choices form the foundation of our health, and the eyes are no exception to this rule. While aging and genetics play a role in many eye conditions, our dietary habits can significantly influence the outcome. By integrating a variety of nutrient-rich foods into our daily diet, we're not just feeding our bodies; we're ensuring our eyes have the best possible tools to function optimally and remain healthy throughout our lives. As we continue our journey into natural vision improvement, let's remain conscious of the fuel we provide our eyes, understanding that our plate's choices directly reflect in our sight.

CHAPTER 21:
THE IMPACT OF
SCREEN TIME

In an era dominated by technology, screens have become an inseparable part of our daily lives. From smartphones and tablets to computers and televisions, digital devices play a pivotal role in how we work, communicate, and unwind. However, this convenience does come at a price. Excessive screen time has emerged as a significant factor impacting our vision. Let's delve into the phenomenon of digital eye strain and explore measures to counteract its effects.

Digital Eye Strain

Digital eye strain, sometimes referred to as computer vision syndrome, encompasses a range of eye discomfort and vision issues resulting from prolonged screen use. The strain isn't just caused by the screens themselves, but also by how we use them. Factors like screen proximity, the duration of use, and even the angle at which we view screens can contribute to this condition.

*Symptoms of Digital Eye Strain: *

- Blurred vision or difficulty focusing
- Dry, irritated, or red eyes
- Headaches, especially after prolonged screen use
- Increased sensitivity to light
- Pain in the neck, shoulders, or back

- Feeling that you cannot keep your eyes open
- General eye discomfort after screen use

Preventive Measures

1. **Proper Screen Placement**: Your computer screen should be 20 to 30 inches away from your eyes. The top of the screen should be at or slightly below your eye level. This reduces the need to tilt your head forward or look down, which can strain the eyes and neck.

2. **Adjust Display Settings**: Increase the text size for easier readability. The contrast between the text and the background should be significant, with black text on a white background being the most comfortable for most people.

3. **Minimize Glare**: Glare from screens and surrounding lights can exacerbate eye strain. Use matte screen protectors and position your screen to avoid reflections from windows or bright lights.

4. **Use the 20-20-20 Rule**: Every 20 minutes, take a 20-second break to look at something 20 feet away. This brief pause can reduce the chances of eye strain significantly.

5. **Blink Regularly**: Blinking refreshes the eye surface. Make a conscious effort to blink more frequently when using digital devices.

6. **Blue Light Filters**: Modern screens emit blue light, which has been implicated in disrupting sleep patterns and contributing to eye strain. Many devices now come with built-in settings or apps that reduce blue light emission, especially in the evenings.

7. **Correct Prescription**: If you wear prescription glasses or contact lenses, ensure they're up to date. Some lenses are specifically designed for screen use, offering magnification or blue light filtering.

8. **Ergonomic Workstations**: Your chair and desk should support a posture where your feet are flat on the ground, and your back is straight. Your screen should be at a position where you don't need to lean forward or look down.

9. **Regular Eye Check-ups**: Ensure you visit an optometrist regularly to address any vision changes or issues promptly.

10. **Reduce Screen Time**: While it's not always feasible given our modern lifestyles, try to limit non-essential screen time. Perhaps pick up a physical book instead of an e-reader or engage in offline hobbies.

11. **Eye Exercises**: Engage in exercises that flex the eye muscles. For instance, roll your eyes in all directions, or focus on a close object and then shift to a distant one repeatedly.

12. **Stay Hydrated**: Drink plenty of water. Proper hydration can prevent dry eyes and support overall eye health.

13. **Adequate Lighting**: The room lighting should be balanced. Too much contrast in brightness between your screen and the surrounding environment can strain the eyes.

In conclusion, while screens have become essential tools in our daily lives, their impact on our eye health is undeniable. By acknowledging the potential risks and adopting preventive measures, we can mitigate the effects of digital eye strain. As with all things related to health, awareness and proactive behavior are our best allies. Embracing a balance between our digital and offline lives will not only benefit our eyes but our overall well-being.

CHAPTER 22: VISUALIZATION AND THE MIND'S EYE

Our eyes serve as windows to the world, capturing countless visuals that shape our perception and experiences. However, it's our mind that processes and interprets these visuals, creating a mental imagery that can be as vivid, if not more so, than the actual scene. This chapter explores the intriguing relationship between visualization and vision, highlighting the powerful role of the mind in vision improvement.

The Power of the Mind in Vision Improvement

Vision is not solely about the mechanical process of light entering the eye and creating an image on the retina. It's an intricate collaboration between the eyes and the brain. Every image that our eyes perceive is translated into neural signals and sent to the brain, which then processes and interprets it. This intimate relationship suggests that the state of our mind can influence the clarity of our vision.

Several studies have indicated that individuals with strong visualization abilities often report better visual clarity. The mind's capacity to visualize can reinforce neural pathways associated with vision, making them more efficient over time.

Moreover, positive visualization can be instrumental in healing and rejuvenation. Athletes, for instance, commonly employ visualization techniques to enhance performance and recover from injuries. Similarly, the act of visualizing clear images can potentially "train" the brain to see more clearly, offering a holistic approach to vision improvement.

Exercises to Strengthen Visualization Skills

1. **Basic Image Holding**:
   * Begin by looking at a simple object, such as a pencil or a coin.
   * Close your eyes and try to see the object in your mind, capturing as much detail as possible.
   * Hold this image for a few moments, then open your eyes and compare the mental image with the actual object.
   * With practice, you'll find that your ability to hold and recall detailed images improves.

2. **Journey Visualization**:
   * Sit comfortably and close your eyes.
   * Imagine you're walking through a familiar path, maybe a route you take daily or a favourite holiday spot.
   * Visualize the details of the journey, including the surroundings, the colours, and the sensations.
   * This exercise not only enhances visualization but also deepens the connection between memory and visual recall.

3. **Dynamic Visualization**:
   * Think of a simple activity, like a bird flying or a leaf floating down a stream.
   * With closed eyes, visualize this activity in your mind, trying to make it as vivid and detailed as possible.
   * Introduce variations: perhaps the bird changes its path, or the leaf gets caught in a whirlpool.

4. **Colour Meditation**:
   * Focus on a specific colour in your mind.
   * Try to fill your entire mental space with that colour, immersing yourself in its hue and depth.
   * Gradually switch to another colour and immerse yourself in

that.

   * This exercise can be calming and enhances colour perception and recall.

5. **Text Visualization**:
   * Read a short paragraph from a book.
   * Close your eyes and try to "read" that paragraph in your mind's eye.
   * This exercise not only bolsters visualization but also improves memory and focus.

6. **Blindfolded Touch**:
   * Blindfold yourself and touch various objects.
   * Try to visualize these objects purely based on touch. This multisensory approach can strengthen the bond between touch and visual recall.

7. **Guided Imagery Sessions**:
   * Listen to guided imagery recordings where a narrator describes serene and detailed scenes, such as a beach during sunset or a bustling marketplace.
   * Such sessions can be deeply relaxing and significantly improve your ability to visualize complex scenes.

In conclusion, the ability to visualize is not just a cognitive luxury but a potent tool that can positively influence our vision. By regularly practicing visualization exercises, we can harness the power of our mind's eye, enhancing our overall visual experience. It reminds us that while our eyes are the instruments, it's our mind that paints the picture, and with a little training, that picture can be as clear and vivid as we desire.

CHAPTER 23: BLINKING: A SIMPLE YET POWERFUL EXERCISER

Blinking, a seemingly insignificant act, is often overlooked in discussions about vision. While it appears to be a simple reflex, blinking plays a crucial role in maintaining the health and clarity of our eyes. It's fascinating how something so instinctual can have profound benefits for our vision. Let's delve deeper into the art of blinking and understand its pivotal role in vision improvement.

The Importance of Frequent, Gentle Blinking

1. Natural Lubrication: Every time you blink, a thin layer of tear film spreads over the cornea, the eye's front surface. This film acts as a natural moisturizer, preventing dryness and ensuring the cornea remains nourished and clear.

2. Protective Barrier: Blinking acts as a defence mechanism. It shields the eyes from potential irritants, such as dust particles and bright lights, by momentarily closing off the external environment.

3. Vision Clarity: The tear film produced by blinking aids in smoothing the corneal surface, which is essential for refraction and visual clarity. When blinking is reduced, such as during prolonged screen usage, it can lead to visual disturbances.

4. Rest and reset: Each blink, though lasting only a fraction of a second, offers a brief respite to the visual system. It's a micro-pause, allowing the eyes and the visual cortex to momentarily reset.

How Blinking Aids in Relaxation and Focus

1. Neural Reset: Blinking is linked with a tiny reset in our brain's default mode network—a network associated with mind-wandering and daydreaming. This neural "refresh" can enhance focus, especially during tasks that require prolonged attention.

2. Reduces Eye Strain: Regular blinking ensures that the eyes remain moist. Dry eyes can lead to a condition known as digital eye strain or computer vision syndrome. Symptoms include redness, burning, blurred vision, and even headaches. By maintaining a steady blinking rhythm, especially during tasks like reading or computer work, one can significantly reduce the risk of eye strain.

3. Mental Breaks: The act of blinking can serve as a subtle cue for the brain to take a micro-break. These minuscule pauses can be refreshing during intensive tasks and can aid in sustained concentration.

4. Mindful Blinking: Being conscious of one's blinking rate can be a form of mindfulness—a mental state where you're fully present and engaged in the moment. Mindful blinking can serve as a grounding exercise, especially when overwhelmed or stressed.

Exercises to Enhance the Blinking Reflex

1. **Conscious Blinking**: Set a timer for two minutes. During this period, blink gently every 3-4 seconds. This exercise can be particularly beneficial if you've been using a screen for a prolonged period.

2. **Blink and Breathe**: Coordinate your blinking with your breathing. As you inhale, keep your eyes open, and as you exhale, blink gently. This exercise not only enhances your blinking reflex but also promotes relaxation.

3. **Blinking Breaks**: If you're engrossed in a task, set reminders to take short blinking breaks. Close your eyes and blink rapidly for 10-15 seconds, then resume your task.

4. **Observation**: Watch others, especially children, and observe their blinking patterns. Children naturally blink more frequently than adults. By emulating this natural rhythm, you can improve your blink rate.

5. **Gentle Shutters**: Instead of a rapid blink, try slowly closing your eyes, holding for a second, and then gently opening them. This extended blink can be particularly soothing if your eyes feel tired or dry.

In conclusion, blinking, while seemingly mundane, holds a powerful secret for vision improvement. By recognizing its importance and ensuring we blink gently and frequently, we can foster better visual health. It's a gentle reminder that sometimes, the simplest actions can have the most profound impacts on our well-being.

CHAPTER 24: THE ROLE OF EMOTIONS IN VISION

Vision, traditionally perceived as a purely physical function, is deeply interconnected with our emotional realm. An intricate dance exists between our eyes and our feelings; our sight can be influenced, sometimes heavily, by our emotional state. This chapter delves into the intertwined relationship between emotions and vision, highlighting the profound impact our inner state can have on our visual clarity.

Exploring the Link Between Emotional Well-Being and Clear Vision

1. Emotional Stress and Eye Strain: Emotional stress, whether acute or chronic, can manifest physically in various ways, including tension in the eye muscles. This tension can lead to eye strain, blurriness, and even headaches. For instance, long periods of intense concentration, anxiety, or worry can lead to reduced blink rate, resulting in dry and strained eyes.

2. Emotional Trauma and Vision Problems: There have been documented cases where individuals experience sudden vision problems after traumatic incidents. While the eyes themselves might be healthy, the psychological trauma can cause visual disturbances, illustrating the profound connection between emotional well-being and vision.

3. Mood and Light Perception: Our emotional state can influence how we perceive brightness and contrast. People in depressive states often describe the world as looking "dimmer" or "greyer." This subjective change in vision underscores the influence of emotions on visual perception.

4. The Relaxation Connection: A relaxed and positive emotional state can enhance visual clarity. When we're calm and happy, our pupil dilation is optimal, eye muscles are relaxed, and we can focus better, leading to sharper vision.

Techniques to Release Emotional Strain for Better Eyesight

1. Emotional Release Meditation:
   * Sit comfortably and close your eyes.
   * Focus on your breathing, taking deep, rhythmic breaths.
   * Visualize any emotional strain or tension as a cloud within you.
   * With each exhale, imagine this cloud dissipating and leaving your body.
   * This visualization can help release emotional blockages, leading to physical relaxation, including in the eyes.

2. Journaling: Writing down your feelings and emotions can be therapeutic. By expressing and acknowledging your emotions, you can reduce the strain they might be imposing on your body, including your eyes.

3. Eye Yoga:
   * Combine traditional eye exercises with emotional release.
   * Focus on an object, then close your eyes and recall a happy memory. Feel the positive emotions as you slowly move your eyes in different directions.
   * Such combined exercises can relieve tension in both the eyes and the mind.

4. Emotional Freedom Techniques (EFT):
   * Also known as tapping, EFT is a process where you tap on

specific acupressure points while vocalizing your feelings.

  * This technique can help in releasing emotional blockages, which can subsequently lead to relaxed and strain-free eyes.

5. Grounding Exercises:
  * When overwhelmed, take a moment to ground yourself.
  * Feel your feet on the ground, touch a nearby object, or focus on ambient sounds.
  * Grounding can pull you out of intense emotional states, reducing their potential impact on your vision.

6. Seek Therapy: Persistent emotional issues and traumas that impact vision might require professional intervention. Therapists can provide tools and techniques to process and release these emotions, leading to holistic well-being, including improved vision.

7. Breathwork:
  * Deep, rhythmic breathing can not only calm the mind but also relax the eye muscles.
  * Incorporate daily sessions of focused breathing, visualizing your eye muscles relaxing with each exhale.

In conclusion, our emotions and vision are inextricably linked. Recognizing and addressing our emotional well-being can lead to clearer, more relaxed eyesight. Vision is not merely a physical function; it's a mirror reflecting our inner state. By nurturing our emotional health, we can indeed pave the way for perfect sight without glasses.

CHAPTER 25: THE 20-20-20 RULE EXPLAINED

In today's digital age, our eyes are incessantly bombarded with screens. Whether for work, leisure, or communication, we find ourselves glued to digital devices, leading to an increasing prevalence of digital eye strain. The 20-20-20 rule has emerged as a simple yet effective strategy to combat this modern-day menace. Let's delve deeper into this rule and discover how it can serve as a protective shield for our eyes in this digital era.

The Modern Approach to Reducing Eye Strain in the Digital Age

**1. What is the 20-20-20 Rule? **
The 20-20-20 rule is straightforward: Every 20 minutes, take a 20-second break and focus your eyes on something at least 20 feet away. This break helps in reducing the strain on the eye muscles that is typically caused by prolonged screen time.

**2. Why is it Needed? **
When we continuously focus on close-up screens, the eye muscles work harder to maintain this near focus. Over time, without breaks, these muscles can become fatigued, leading to symptoms like blurred vision, dry eyes, headaches, and even neck or shoulder pain. The 20-20-20 rule serves as a regular respite for these muscles, allowing them to relax and rejuvenate.

3. The Science Behind the Rule
Focusing on distant objects requires less effort from our eye muscles than focusing on close-up objects. By redirecting our focus to something far away, we effectively give our eyes a mini workout session, stretching and relaxing the muscles, thereby reducing the risk of accommodation spasm, a condition where the eye muscles find it challenging to focus on distant objects after prolonged close work.

Practical Ways to Implement the Rule in Daily Life

**1. Set Timed Reminders: **
One of the most effective ways to incorporate the 20-20-20 rule is by setting timed reminders. Whether through a phone alarm, a desktop app, or smartwatch vibrations, regular reminders will ensure you don't get too engrossed in your work and forget to give your eyes a break.

**2. Use Your Environment: **
Find a window or a distant object in your vicinity that you can focus on during your breaks. It could be a tree, a building, or any other distant object. The act of looking outside can also mentally refresh you.

**3. Pair with Physical Movement: **
Combine the 20-20-20 rule with a quick stretch. Stand up, move around, and take deep breaths. This not only benefits your eyes but also prevents other sedentary-related issues like stiff joints or poor circulation.

**4. Blink More Often: **
During your 20-second break, make a conscious effort to blink more frequently. Blinking helps moisten the eyes, reducing the dryness and irritation associated with prolonged screen time.

**5. Adjust Your Workspace: **
Ensure that your screen is at eye level and about an arm's length away. This positioning reduces the strain on both your eyes and

neck. Also, consider adjusting the brightness and contrast of your screen to ensure it's comfortable to look at.

**6. Natural Light Advantage: **
If possible, position your workspace near a source of natural light. Natural light is gentler on the eyes than artificial lighting. During your 20-second breaks, look outside and focus on natural elements, which can be soothing for the eyes.

**7. Use Technology Aids: **
There are various apps and software available that remind users to take breaks based on the 20-20-20 rule. These tools can be especially helpful for those who find it challenging to remember to take breaks on their own.

**8. Educate and Advocate: **
Spread awareness about the 20-20-20 rule among colleagues, friends, and family. Encouraging group breaks can make adherence to the rule more enjoyable and social.

In conclusion, the 20-20-20 rule is a testament to the fact that sometimes, the simplest solutions can be the most effective. In an era dominated by screens, this rule stands as an easily accessible tool that everyone, irrespective of age or profession, can employ to safeguard their vision. As we navigate the digital age, it's crucial to remember that our eyes, like any other part of our body, need regular breaks to function at their best. Adopting the 20-20-20 rule is a small yet significant step towards ensuring perfect sight without glasses.

CHAPTER 26: EYE YOGA: MOVEMENT AND FLEXIBILITY

While yoga, with its myriad poses and deep breaths, has traditionally been associated with flexibility of the body and tranquillity of the mind, its principles can extend to one of our most vital organs: the eyes. Given the eyes' essential role and the strain they undergo daily, they deserve dedicated care. Eye yoga, drawing inspiration from age-old yoga principles, offers exercises that promote ocular health and flexibility. Let's dive deep into the realm of eye yoga and understand its significance.

Introducing Eye Exercises Inspired by Yoga Principles

1. Palming:
Begin by rubbing your palms together until they feel warm. Close your eyes and gently place your palms over your eyelids, ensuring no pressure is exerted on the eyeballs. Feel the warmth seep through, relaxing your eyes. Take deep breaths and enjoy this restful pose for a few minutes. It's akin to the 'Savasana' or corpse pose for your eyes.

2. Sideways Viewing:
Sit in a comfortable position with legs crossed. Without moving your head, look to your extreme left and then to your extreme right. Repeat this horizontal movement 5-10 times. This exercise helps improve peripheral vision and strengthens the muscles that control the eye's side-to-side movements.

3. Up and Down Viewing:
Maintaining a straight head position, focus your eyes on a point overhead and then slowly shift your gaze to a point down towards the floor. Repeat this vertical movement 5-10 times, allowing the eye muscles to stretch and contract.

4. Diagonal Viewing:
Start by looking up to the top-left corner and then diagonally down to the bottom-right corner. After a few repetitions, switch to looking from the top-right corner to the bottom-left corner. This diagonal movement enhances the flexibility of eye muscles.

5. Front and Distant Viewing:
Focus on a close object for a few seconds, then shift your gaze to a distant object. This near and far viewing exercise helps in adjusting focus and strengthens the ciliary muscles of the eyes.

6. Rotational Viewing:
Imagine a clock in front of you. Focus your gaze on the 12 o'clock position, then move to 1 o'clock, 2 o'clock, and so on, tracing the clock's periphery. Once you complete the circle, reverse the direction. This rotational exercise improves the eyes' ability to track moving objects smoothly.

7. Blinking:
Sitting comfortably, blink your eyes rapidly 10-15 times, ensuring full lid closure with each blink. After a set, close your eyes and relax. Rapid blinking lubricates the eyes and offers a refreshing break, especially for those who spend long hours in front of screens.

Benefits of Maintaining Ocular Muscle Flexibility

1. Reduced Eye Strain:
Regular eye exercises, by promoting muscle flexibility, can alleviate the symptoms of eye strain. Eye yoga provides a balanced workout for the various muscles that control eye movements, ensuring they remain supple and responsive.

2. Enhanced Focus Adjustment:
The ability to shift focus from near to distant objects and vice versa is crucial. Eye yoga exercises, like front and distant viewing, train the eyes to adjust focus more efficiently.

3. Improved Blood Circulation:
Like any other muscles, the ocular muscles benefit from increased blood flow, which delivers essential nutrients. Eye yoga helps in enhancing circulation, ensuring the eyes remain nourished.

4. Counteracting Digital Eye Strain:
In our tech-driven world, digital eye strain is rampant. Eye yoga offers a holistic approach to counteract the effects of prolonged screen exposure, promoting relaxation and reducing dryness.

5. Enhanced Visual Agility:
Visual agility, the eyes' ability to track moving objects smoothly, is vital for tasks like reading or sports. Exercises like rotational viewing enhance this capability.

6. Preventive Care:
While eye yoga boosts eye health, it also serves as a preventive measure, potentially delaying the onset of certain vision-related issues that arise from muscle rigidity and continuous strain.

In conclusion, eye yoga, with its array of exercises rooted in time-tested yoga principles, offers a holistic approach to eye care. It reminds us that the eyes, just like any other part of our body, require regular exercise and care. Embracing eye yoga can pave the way to better visual health, ensuring that the quest for perfect sight without glasses is not just a dream but a reachable reality.

CHAPTER 27: CENTRAL AND PERIPHERAL VISION

In the intricate choreography of sight, two main players stand out: central and peripheral vision. Both are fundamental, yet each plays a unique role, weaving together a complete picture of the world around us. Understanding their differences and nurturing both forms of vision can pave the way to more holistic eyesight. This chapter dives deep into the realms of central and peripheral vision, illuminating their distinct roles and offering exercises to harmonize and enhance their functions.

Understanding the Difference and Their Roles

1. Central Vision:
Central vision, also known as foveal vision, refers to the direct line of sight. It's the vision you use when you focus on a specific object, person, or detail. When reading, threading a needle, or recognizing a face, it's your central vision at work.

- **Role**: Central vision is responsible for sharpness, clarity, and colour perception. It enables us to perform tasks that require detail, precision, and recognition.

2. Peripheral Vision:
Peripheral vision encompasses the wider field of vision that lies outside the central gaze, often referred to as side vision. While not as sharp as central vision, it's crucial for detecting motion

and spatial awareness.

- **Role**: This form of vision is vital for detecting movements in the broader visual field, aiding in navigation and ensuring safety. For example, when you spot a car approaching from the side while crossing the road or sense someone approaching from behind, that's your peripheral vision in action.

The beautiful dance between central and peripheral vision gives us a comprehensive visual experience. While the central vision narrows down on details, the peripheral vision ensures we're aware of the bigger picture, the context in which those details exist.

Exercises to Enhance and Balance Both Forms of Vision

1. Central Vision Focus Exercise:

- **Target Practice**: Place a small target, like a letter or a picture, on a wall. Stand at a distance, gradually focusing on the target. Try to see the details clearly. Move closer or farther away, challenging your central vision to adjust and focus.

2. Peripheral Vision Awareness Exercise:

- **Wide Field Viewing**: Sit comfortably and, while keeping your head still, stretch out your arms to your sides. Wiggle your fingers and, using only your eyes, try to detect the movement. Gradually bring your arms forward while continuing the wiggling and determine the point at which your fingers come into clear view. This exercise broadens your awareness of the peripheral field.

3. Central-Peripheral Switch:

- **Focus Shift**: Place two objects at different distances in the same line of sight, one close and one far. Focus on the closer object, taking in its details, then quickly shift your focus to the distant object. This rapid switch between central and peripheral vision sharpens both and improves the eye's ability to adjust focus quickly.

4. Peripheral Motion Detection:

- **Passing Object**: While focusing on a central point, have someone pass an object, like a ball, from one side to the other in your peripheral field. Without moving your central gaze, try to detect and track the object using only your peripheral vision. This enhances motion detection capabilities.

5. Expanding the Visual Field:

- **Peripheral Drawing**: On a large sheet of paper, draw or pin images at the far edges. While focusing on a central point, try to identify and 'see' the images at the periphery. The goal is to expand and be more aware of the boundaries of your peripheral vision.

6. Balancing Exercise:

- **Walking the Line**: Draw a straight line on the ground. While walking on the line, focusing on keeping your feet aligned, use your peripheral vision to detect any obstacles placed on either side. This exercise helps in balancing the use of central vision for precision and peripheral vision for awareness.

In conclusion, both central and peripheral vision are invaluable assets to our visual experience. Recognizing their distinct roles and ensuring they are both honed and balanced can lead to richer, clearer, and more dynamic sight. As we aim for perfect sight without glasses, giving due importance to every facet of our vision becomes imperative. Through understanding and exercises, we can ensure that both our focused gaze and wide-eyed awareness are in perfect harmony.

CHAPTER 28: IMPROVING NIGHT VISION

For many, the cloak of the night brings with it challenges in visual clarity. Street signs become blurred, familiar paths appear unfamiliar, and the once vibrant colours of the day fade into indistinguishable shades. Night vision, or our ability to see in low-light conditions, is crucial not just for nightly activities but also for ensuring safety during tasks like driving. This chapter sheds light on the causes of poor night vision and offers holistic strategies and exercises to help enhance visual acuity when daylight fades.

Causes of Poor Night Vision

1. **Age**: As we age, the lenses in our eyes become less transparent, reducing the amount of light that reaches the retina. This natural process can diminish night vision.

2. **Vitamin A Deficiency**: Vitamin A plays a vital role in producing rhodopsin, a pigment found in the eyes that aids night vision. A deficiency can led to challenges seeing in the dark.

3. **Cataracts**: The clouding of the lens, commonly known as cataracts, can scatter incoming light, making it challenging to see clearly in low-light situations.

4. **Certain Medications**: Some medications can have side

effects that impair night vision. Always check with your healthcare provider if you notice any changes after starting a new medication.

5. **Lack of Exposure to Darkness**: Spending extended periods in brightly lit areas can diminish the eyes' ability to adapt to darkness quickly.

Strategies and Exercises to Enhance Visual Clarity in Low Light

1. **Nutrition for Night Vision**:
   - **Vitamin A-Rich Foods**: Incorporating foods rich in Vitamin A, such as carrots, sweet potatoes, and dark leafy greens, can support better night vision.
   - **Zinc**: Found in beans, nuts, and meat, zinc aids Vitamin A in producing melanin, a protective pigment in the eyes.
   - **Antioxidants**: Berries, grapes, and spinach are packed with antioxidants that can protect eyes from free radicals and improve overall eye health.

2. **Adaptation Practice**:
   - **Switching Environments**: Regularly switch between well-lit and dimly lit rooms. This practice helps the eyes adapt more swiftly to changing light conditions, enhancing their responsiveness during transitions from light to dark.

3. **Peripheral Gaze**:
   - In low light, the peripheral retina, which is rich in rod cells (sensitive to dim light), becomes more active. Practice focusing on objects using your peripheral vision. This not only improves night vision but also enhances spatial awareness in the dark.

4. **Blinking Exercise**:
   - Blinking refreshes the eye surface. In dim environments, practice gentle, deliberate blinking. This exercise can help clear the visual field and enhance focus in low light.

5. **Eye Palming for Relaxation**:

- Warm your palms by rubbing them together. Close your eyes and gently cup them with your palms, ensuring no pressure on the eyeballs. The warmth and darkness allow the eyes to relax and can assist in better adaptation to low light environments.

6. **Avoid Direct Light Exposure**:
   - If you're transitioning from a bright environment to a darker one, avoid looking directly at strong light sources. This ensures that the eyes remain sensitive and adaptable to the dimmer surroundings.

7. **Contrast Training**:
   - Practice focusing on objects against contrasting backgrounds. In a dimly lit room, place dark objects against lighter backdrops and vice versa. Try to discern the details of the object. This exercise strengthens the eyes' ability to pick out details in varying light conditions.

8. **Limit Screen Time Before Night Activities**:
   - Prolonged exposure to bright screens can reduce the eyes' efficiency in transitioning to the dark. If you know you'll be navigating in low light, such as driving at night, reduce screen time beforehand.

In conclusion, night vision, like other aspects of sight, can be nurtured and enhanced with awareness, practice, and care. By understanding the causes of its impairment and actively engaging in strategies and exercises, one can navigate the world of twilight with greater confidence and clarity. Perfect sight without glasses isn't just a daytime endeavour—it extends into the realm of moonlit nights and starry skies. By shining a light on the challenges and solutions of night vision, we ensure that every moment, day or night, is seen with clarity and brilliance.

CHAPTER 29: THE IMPORTANCE OF PROPER LIGHTING

The sun dapples through the leaves, casting a gentle glow on the pages of a book, or the harsh fluorescent lights at the office cause an unwanted glare on the computer screen — light, in its myriad forms, plays a paramount role in how we perceive the world. Not only does the right lighting accentuate the beauty of our surroundings, but it also significantly influences our visual health. This chapter delves into the types of light and their effects on vision, offering guidance on how to optimize lighting for various activities to protect and enhance our eyesight.

Analysing the Types of Light and Their Impacts on Vision

1. **Natural Light (Sunlight)**:
   - **Pros**: Sunlight offers a balanced spectrum of colours, making it the most comfortable and healthiest form of light for our eyes. It enhances clarity, reduces eye strain, and elevates mood.
   - **Cons**: Direct exposure to intense sunlight can harm the eyes due to ultraviolet (UV) rays, potentially leading to conditions like cataracts.

2. **Incandescent Bulbs**:
   - **Pros**: These bulbs produce warm, yellowish light that can be easy on the eyes and create a cosy ambiance.
   - **Cons**: They can be inefficient in terms of energy

consumption and may not be ideal for tasks requiring precise colour recognition.

3. **Fluorescent Lights**:
   - **Pros**: They're energy-efficient and provide bright illumination, suitable for large spaces like offices.
   - **Cons**: The blueish hue of some fluorescent lights can be harsh on the eyes, leading to eye strain and glare. The flickering, often imperceptible, can also be a source of visual discomfort.

4. **LED Lights**:
   - **Pros**: LEDs are highly energy-efficient, long-lasting, and can be designed to offer various colour temperatures, from cool to warm.
   - **Cons**: Blue light emission from certain LEDs can potentially contribute to eye strain and interfere with sleep patterns if used late into the night.

Tips for Optimizing Lighting for Reading, Work, and Relaxation

1. **Reading**:
   - **Angle and Position**: Position the light source behind you and direct it onto your reading material. Avoid placing it directly behind the reading material to prevent casting shadows.
   - **Brightness**: Ensure the light is bright enough to illuminate the text clearly without being overpowering.
   - **Natural Light**: Whenever possible, opt for reading in natural light. Position your reading chair near a window but be cautious of direct sunlight exposure.

2. **Work (Especially Digital Work)**:
   - **Ambient Lighting**: Ensure that the entire room is well-lit to prevent sharp contrasts which can lead to eye strain. Dim rooms with bright screens are a recipe for visual discomfort.
   - **Task Lighting**: For non-digital tasks, use adjustable desk lamps that can focus light directly where you need it.
   - **Reduce Glare**: Position computer screens to avoid

reflections from windows and lights. Consider using matte screen protectors.

3. **Relaxation**:
   - **Warm Lighting**: opt for warmer, dimmer lights to create a calming ambiance. Incandescent bulbs or warm LEDs are great choices.
   - **Avoid Blue Light Before Bed**: Blue light can interfere with the production of melatonin, a hormone essential for sleep. If you use devices before bed, consider blue light filters or "night mode" settings.

4. **General Tips**:
   - **Layered Lighting**: Combine different light sources to cater to various tasks and moods. For instance, use ambient lighting for overall room illumination, task lighting for specific activities, and accent lighting to highlight decor.
   - **Adjustable Brightness**: Use dimmer switches or adjustable lamps to change the brightness according to the time of day and activity.
   - **Protect from Direct Sunlight**: While natural light is beneficial, direct exposure can be harmful. Use curtains or blinds to control the intensity of sunlight entering a room.

In conclusion, while light illuminates our world, enabling us to see and appreciate its beauty, it's crucial to ensure that this illumination is optimized for our visual well-being. Proper lighting is an often overlooked yet crucial aspect of natural vision improvement. By being mindful of the type and quality of light we expose our eyes to, we can foster clearer vision and reduce the risk of strain, fatigue, and other visual ailments. As we journey towards perfect sight without glasses, let's shine the right light on our path, making every step brighter and clearer.

CHAPTER 30: CORRECTING DOUBLE VISION AND STRABISMUS

Within the complex tapestry of visual anomalies, double vision (diplopia) and strabismus stand out as conditions that not only affect the clarity of sight but also the alignment of the eyes. This chapter explores these two intertwined conditions, shedding light on their origins and introducing natural techniques and exercises that can aid in their correction.

Understanding the Causes of These Conditions

1. **Double Vision (Diplopia)**:
   - **Definition**: Diplopia, or double vision, is a condition where a person sees two images of a single object. This can be horizontally, vertically, or diagonally displaced.
   - **Causes**:
      - **Muscle Imbalance**: A disparity in the strength and coordination of the eye muscles can lead to misalignment, resulting in double vision.
      - **Lens Problems**: Conditions like cataracts can sometimes cause diplopia.
      - **Nervous System Issues**: Diseases affecting the nervous system, like multiple sclerosis or strokes, can impair the nerves controlling the eye muscles.

- **Trauma**: Direct injury to the eyes or surrounding structures can lead to diplopia.

2. **Strabismus**:
   - **Definition**: Often referred to as "crossed eyes" or "wall-eyed," strabismus is a misalignment of the eyes, where they do not look in the same direction simultaneously.
   - **Causes**:
      - **Congenital Factors**: Some individuals are born with strabismus due to genetic or developmental reasons.
      - **Loss of Vision**: An eye that cannot see well might drift and become misaligned.
      - **Nerve or Muscle Damage**: Injuries or diseases can affect the muscles or nerves, leading to strabismus.
      - **Refractive Errors**: Significant differences in prescription between the eyes can sometimes lead to strabismus.

Natural Techniques and Exercises to Aid in Correction

1. **Eye Muscle Strengthening**:
   - **Pencil Pushups**: Holding a pencil (or a similar object) vertically, focus on the tip and slowly move it towards your nose, keeping your eyes converged on the target. When you see double, stop and focus until a single image is seen, then continue. Do this several times a day.

   - **Brock String Exercise**: Using a long string with three coloured beads spaced out, focus on each bead starting from the closest to the farthest, ensuring that you see only one bead while the others appear double. This helps with convergence and divergence.

2. **Gaze Shifting**:
   - **Horizontal Gaze Shift**: Place two stickers or objects at eye level, one close and one farther away. Shift your gaze from one to the other, spending a few seconds focusing on each. This can improve coordination between the eyes.

- **Vertical Gaze Shift**: Similar to the horizontal exercise, but place one sticker/object above eye level and the other below. Shift your gaze up and down.

3. **Patch Therapy**:
   - **Alternating Eye Patching**: By covering the stronger or dominant eye for a specific time, the weaker or misaligned eye is encouraged to work harder. This can gradually help in aligning the eyes. Always consult with an optometrist before starting patch therapy.

4. **Focus on Near and Far Objects**:
   - Spend time focusing on close-up tasks, like reading, followed by looking at distant objects outside. This transition can help in training the eyes to work together.

5. **Relaxation Techniques**:
   - Often, strabismus or diplopia can be exacerbated by stress. Techniques such as deep breathing, meditation, and visualization can help relax both the mind and the ocular muscles.

6. **Vision Therapy**:
   - Under the guidance of a trained optometrist, vision therapy employs various tools and techniques to improve eye coordination, convergence, and reduce strabismus and double vision.

In conclusion, while double vision and strabismus present their unique challenges, understanding their causes lays the foundation for embarking on a path of natural correction. By integrating exercises that bolster eye muscle strength and coordination, one can gradually witness improvements in alignment and vision. As always, individual experiences may vary, and it's crucial to consult with a vision care professional before beginning any new regimen. As we aspire for perfect sight without glasses, let's remember that patience, consistency, and holistic well-being are integral to the journey.

CHAPTER 31: OVERCOMING EYE FATIGUE

Eye fatigue, also known as asthenopia, is a common yet often overlooked condition in the modern world. With the prevalence of screens, inadequate lighting, and prolonged visual tasks, our eyes frequently bear the brunt of our demanding lifestyles. This chapter will help you understand the signs of eye fatigue, delve into its causes, and equip you with strategies to rejuvenate tired eyes and prevent future occurrences.

Recognizing Symptoms and Causes of Eye Fatigue

1. **Symptoms of Eye Fatigue**:
   - **Blurry or Double Vision**: After prolonged focus, especially on digital devices, vision can become blurred or even doubled.
   - **Sore or Itchy Eyes**: A sensation of discomfort, itching, or even burning in the eyes.
   - **Heavy Eyelids**: Feeling like it requires effort to keep the eyelids open.
   - **Increased Sensitivity to Light**: Finding bright lights or even normal daylight too glaring.
   - **Headaches**: Particularly those centred around the temples or forehead.
   - **Difficulty Concentrating**: A decreased ability to focus on tasks.
   - **Dry or Watery Eyes**: An imbalance in tear production,

leading to either excessive dryness or watering.

2. **Causes of Eye Fatigue**:

   - **Prolonged Screen Time**: Extended periods on computers, smartphones, or televisions can strain the eyes, mainly due to blue light emission and reduced blink rate.

   - **Inadequate Lighting**: Straining to read or work in poorly lit conditions can overexert the eye muscles.

   - **Extended Focus on Close-up Tasks**: Activities like reading, sewing, or drawing for extended periods without breaks can lead to fatigue.

   - **Underlying Vision Issues**: Unaddressed or incorrectly addressed refractive errors like myopia, hyperopia, or astigmatism can add to the strain.

   - **Environmental Factors**: Dry air, dust, or allergens can irritate the eyes, leading to fatigue.

   - **Incorrect Ergonomics**: If your work setup isn't optimized — for instance, a computer screen positioned too high or too low — it can cause unnecessary strain.

Strategies for Rejuvenation and Prevention

1. **The 20-20-20 Rule**: Every 20 minutes, take a 20-second break and look at something 20 feet away. This simple habit helps to reset your focus and give your eye muscles a much-needed break.

2. **Proper Lighting**: Ensure that your workspace is well-lit, preferably with natural light. If that's not possible, opt for warm, ambient lighting rather than a single harsh source.

3. **Blink Regularly**: Blinking naturally lubricates the eyes. Make a conscious effort to blink more frequently, especially when using digital devices.

4. **Adjust Screen Brightness and Use Blue Light Filters**: Your screen's brightness should match the lighting of your environment. Using built-in or third-party blue light filters can

also reduce the strain caused by prolonged screen exposure.

5. **Ergonomic Setup**: Ensure that your screen is at eye level, and about an arm's length away. This reduces the angle of gaze and prevents undue strain on the neck and eyes.

6. **Eye Exercises**:
   - **Palming**: Rub your hands together to generate warmth and gently cup them over your closed eyes without pressing. The darkness and warmth help to relax the eyes.
   - **Rolling**: Close your eyes and gently roll them in a circular motion, first clockwise and then counter-clockwise.
   - **Focus Shifting**: Regularly shift your focus from near to far objects to exercise the eye muscles.

7. **Stay Hydrated**: Drink plenty of water. Hydration aids in tear production, which keeps the eyes moist and refreshed.

8. **Limit Screen Time**: Set limits on non-essential screen time, especially before bed. This not only helps your eyes but can also improve sleep quality.

9. **Use Artificial Tears**: If your eyes feel dry, over-the-counter lubricating eye drops can provide relief. However, avoid over-relying on them and consult an optometrist if you find the need to use them frequently.

10. **Regular Eye Check-ups**: Ensure you get your eyes checked regularly. Addressing even minor vision issues can significantly reduce the strain on your eyes.

In conclusion, eye fatigue, while common, shouldn't be accepted as an inevitable part of modern life. With awareness of its causes and proactive measures, we can ensure our eyes remain refreshed and ready to tackle the visual demands of our world. Remember, our eyes are not just windows to the soul but also our primary means of interacting with the world around us. Let's give them the care they truly deserve.

CHAPTER 32: THE ROLE OF SLEEP IN VISION HEALTH

Sleep, often termed as the body's natural recharge mechanism, plays a pivotal role in maintaining overall health, and our vision is no exception to this rule. Restful sleep has myriad benefits, many of which directly and indirectly affect our eyes. This chapter will delve into the profound connection between sleep and vision health and offer insights on how to optimize sleep for the sake of our eyes.

How Quality Sleep Impacts Eye Health

1. **Cellular Repair and Regeneration**: Just as the body uses sleep as a time to repair damaged cells, the eyes, too, undergo a process of healing and restoration. During the deepest stages of sleep, cell growth and repair occur, helping to mend the minor damages the eyes may have experienced during the day, like exposure to harmful UV rays or screen time.

2. **Eye Lubrication**: The consistency and distribution of the tear film that lubricates our eyes are improved with sleep. A good night's sleep ensures that our eyes are adequately moistened, preventing dryness and irritation.

3. **Clearing Out Debris**: Throughout the day, small debris and particles can get into our eyes. Sleep provides the eyes an opportunity to clear out this potential irritant, reducing the risk

of infections or inflammation.

4. **Reducing Eye Strain**: Prolonged wakefulness, especially in the digital age where screens are omnipresent, can result in eye strain. Sleep gives the eyes the necessary break from continuous exposure and helps in reducing the cumulative effects of visual strain.

5. **Improved Focus and Sharpness**: Chronic sleep deprivation can lead to blurred vision. Quality sleep helps maintain the eyes' ability to focus and ensures visual clarity.

6. **Emotional Well-being**: Lack of sleep can lead to stress, anxiety, and mood disorders. Emotional well-being is intrinsically linked to vision, as stress can exacerbate conditions like blurry vision or eye twitching. Hence, proper sleep indirectly supports vision health by maintaining emotional balance.

Tips for Ensuring a Restful Night for the Benefit of the Eyes

1. **Consistent Sleep Schedule**: Sticking to a regular sleep schedule, even on weekends, helps set your body's internal clock, leading to better sleep quality. Aim for 7-9 hours nightly.

2. **Screen-Free Time**: Blue light from digital devices can hinder the production of melatonin, a hormone responsible for sleep. Establish a habit of disconnecting from screens at least an hour before bedtime.

3. **Optimal Sleep Environment**: Your bedroom should be cool, dark, and quiet. Consider using blackout curtains, earplugs, or a white noise machine if necessary. An ideal room temperature lies somewhere around 60-67 degrees Fahrenheit (15-19 degrees Celsius).

4. **Limit Caffeine and Alcohol**: Both can interfere with sleep. Limit their consumption, especially in the evening hours.

5. **Bedtime Ritual**: Calming activities, like reading (preferably

a physical book), practicing deep breathing, or gentle stretching, can signal the body that it's time to wind down.

6. **Proper Pillow and Mattress**: Ensure that your pillow and mattress support your head, neck, and spine adequately. An uncomfortable sleep position can not only disrupt sleep but also strain the muscles around the eyes.

7. **Be Mindful of Diet**: Consuming a large meal or heavy, spicy foods right before bed can lead to discomfort and indigestion, disrupting sleep. If hungry, opt for a light, healthy snack.

8. **Eye Relaxation Techniques**: Incorporate eye relaxation exercises into your bedtime routine. Gentle palming or eyelid massages can help soothe strained eyes and prepare them for rest.

9. **Stay Hydrated**: Drink enough water throughout the day but reduce intake right before bedtime to minimize middle-of-the-night bathroom trips.

10. **Seek Medical Advice for Persistent Sleep Issues**: If you find yourself struggling with sleep regularly, it might be worth consulting a sleep specialist. Conditions like sleep apnea can severely disrupt sleep quality and have ramifications for eye health.

In conclusion, sleep is not merely a luxury but a necessity, especially when it comes to maintaining the health of our eyes. By prioritizing sleep and adopting habits that foster restful nights, we do more than just banish under-eye circles; we provide our eyes with the recuperative environment they need to serve us well each day. A commitment to sleep is, in essence, a commitment to clearer, healthier vision.

CHAPTER 33: THE IMPACT OF BLUE LIGHT

Blue light, a high-energy visible (HEV) light, has recently come into the spotlight due to its omnipresence in our digital world. Found naturally in sunlight, it also emanates from our digital screens, such as smartphones, computers, and LED televisions. Though an essential component of the light spectrum, prolonged exposure to artificial blue light from digital devices has raised concerns about its effect on our eye health and overall well-being. This chapter will explore these effects and provide guidance on how to mitigate potential harms.

Delving into the Effects of Digital Screens on Our Eyes

1. **Digital Eye Strain**: Prolonged exposure to screens, coupled with the high concentration of blue light they emit, can lead to what's commonly referred to as digital eye strain or computer vision syndrome. Symptoms include dry eyes, headaches, blurry vision, and difficulty focusing.

2. **Potential Retinal Damage**: Some studies suggest that excessive exposure to blue light might lead to retinal cell damage. Over time, this damage could contribute to age-related macular degeneration, a condition leading to vision loss.

3. **Disrupted Circadian Rhythm**: Blue light has been shown to suppress the secretion of melatonin more than other types of

light. Melatonin is a hormone responsible for regulating sleep. Thus, using screens, especially before bedtime, can interfere with the body's natural sleep-wake cycle, leading to sleep disturbances.

4. **Potential Link to Cataract Development**: Preliminary research has hinted at a connection between prolonged blue light exposure and an increased risk of developing cataracts, although more extensive studies are needed to confirm this link.

5. **Increased Sensitivity to Light**: Overexposure to blue light might make individuals more sensitive to all light types, a condition known as photophobia.

Recommendations for Minimizing Blue Light Exposure

1. **Follow the 20-20-20 Rule**: This rule is a simple yet effective way to give your eyes a break. Every 20 minutes, take a 20-second break and focus on something at least 20 feet away. This brief pause can help reduce eye strain.

2. **Screen Filters**: There are numerous over-the-counter blue light filters available for screens. These filters can be easily attached to the display of your devices, cutting down the amount of blue light they emit.

3. **Wear Blue Light Blocking Glasses**: These specialized glasses have lenses that reduce or block blue light from entering your eyes. They can be particularly beneficial for individuals who spend considerable time in front of screens, whether for work or leisure.

4. **Adjust Screen Brightness and Contrast**: Your screen's brightness should match the ambient light level in your environment. Additionally, increasing the contrast can reduce the strain on your eyes.

5. **Maintain an Optimal Distance**: Keeping screens at an arm's length distance, or at least 20 inches away, can reduce the

intensity of blue light reaching the eyes.

6. **Limit Screen Time Before Bed**: To preserve your sleep cycle, avoid screens for at least an hour before bedtime. If this isn't possible, consider using "night mode" or "warm light" settings on devices, which reduce blue light emissions.

7. **Regular Eye Exams**: Regular check-ups with an optometrist can help in early detection of any potential issues related to blue light exposure. Moreover, they can provide personalized advice based on your screen habits.

8. **Blink Frequently**: Blinking moisturizes the eyes, reducing dryness and irritation. Make a conscious effort to blink more often when using digital devices.

9. **Ensure Proper Lighting**: Using screens in a well-lit environment reduces the contrast between the screen and the surrounding area, minimizing eye strain. Avoid using devices in the dark.

10. **Stay Informed**: As research on blue light's effects continues, it's crucial to stay updated. Adjust your habits as new findings emerge to ensure optimal eye health.

In summation, while blue light is an unavoidable aspect of modern life, understanding its implications and taking preventive measures can help in safeguarding our vision. By being proactive and incorporating the above recommendations, one can enjoy the benefits of technology without compromising eye health.

CHAPTER 34: KEEPING THE EYES ACTIVE: A LIFELONG JOURNEY

The human body is designed for movement. Just as our limbs require exercise and our minds crave stimulation, our eyes, too, need regular activity to stay healthy and sharp. Eye activity, both intentional and incidental, plays a vital role in maintaining vision clarity. This chapter delves into the importance of nurturing active eyes and fostering vision habits that stand the test of time.

The Significance of Regular Eye Movement and Exercise

1. **Promotes Blood Circulation**: Regular eye movement enhances blood circulation to the eyes, ensuring a steady supply of essential nutrients and oxygen. This increased circulation is pivotal for repairing daily wear and tear and reducing the risk of degenerative conditions.

2. **Stimulates Eye Muscles**: The eyes house six intricate muscles that control their movement. Keeping these muscles engaged prevents them from becoming stiff or weak over time, much like how body exercises maintain muscle tone.

3. **Relieves Eye Strain**: Intentional eye exercises can alleviate the strain caused by prolonged periods of fixed focus, such as reading or screen time. Regular breaks and exercises can refresh the eyes and minimize fatigue.

4. **Improves Focus and Flexibility**: Regular eye activity can enhance the eyes' ability to shift focus between near and distant objects. This adaptability is often termed 'accommodation' and is vital for tasks like driving, where one needs to constantly adjust their gaze.

5. **Supports Vision Acuity**: Engaging in a regimen of eye exercises can, over time, contribute to clearer vision by training the eyes to work optimally.

Maintaining Good Vision Habits Throughout Life

1. **Integrate Eye Breaks**: Whether you're studying, working, or enjoying a movie, practice the 20-20-20 rule. Every 20 minutes, glance at an object 20 feet away for 20 seconds. This simple habit reduces eye strain and breaks the monotony of a fixed gaze.

2. **Adopt Eye Exercises**: Integrate exercises into your daily routine. This can be as simple as focusing on a nearby object and then a distant one, repeating several times. Alternatively, trace imaginary figures with your gaze, or practice moving your eyes in different directions without turning your head.

3. **Stay Physically Active**: General physical activity also benefits the eyes. Regular exercise improves blood circulation throughout the body, including the eyes. Moreover, outdoor activities expose the eyes to varying distances and light conditions, which is invigorating for them.

4. **Protect Your Eyes**: Always shield your eyes from harmful UV rays by wearing sunglasses when outdoors. When involved in sports or activities with potential eye hazards, wear protective eyewear.

5. **Maintain a Balanced Diet**: Nutritional intake profoundly impacts eye health. Incorporate foods rich in Vitamin A, C, E, and minerals like zinc. Omega-3 fatty acids, found in fish, are

known to reduce the risk of age-related vision issues.

6. **Stay Hydrated**: Drink plenty of water to ensure your eyes remain moist and cleansed from impurities.

7. **Limit Screen Time**: While screens have become integral to our lives, it's essential to moderate their use. Beyond adopting the 20-20-20 rule, ensure your workspace is well-lit and consider using screen protectors that filter out blue light.

8. **Prioritize Sleep**: A good night's rest is vital. Sleep allows the eyes to repair and rejuvenate. It clears out debris and ensures the eyes are fresh and ready for the next day.

9. **Regular Check-ups**: Even if you have perfect vision, get regular eye check-ups. They can detect early signs of potential issues, ensuring timely intervention.

10. **Stay Curious and Engaged**: Stimulate your visual senses by exploring new environments, reading, or taking up hobbies like puzzles, drawing, or painting. Such activities keep the eyes active, and the brain's visual centre engaged.

To truly honour our vision, we must acknowledge that eye care is not a one-time endeavour but a lifelong commitment. It's not just about reacting to problems but proactively ensuring that our eyes receive the care and stimulation they need. By adopting and maintaining these habits, we can ensure that our eyes remain active, healthy, and clear, allowing us to savour the visual wonders of the world throughout our lives.

Part IV: Advanced Techniques and Exercises

CHAPTER 35: ADVANCED PALMING TECHNIQUES

Palming, an age-old relaxation technique, has long been recognized for its profound effects on visual health. Rooted in the belief that eyes rejuvenate and heal best in complete darkness, palming not only offers a respite to strained eyes but can also be a gateway to deeper relaxation and potent visualizations. This chapter explores advanced methods to elevate the traditional palming practice, offering a deeper understanding and enhanced benefits.

The Basics of Palming

Before diving into advanced techniques, it's essential to reiterate the foundation of palming.

1. Sit comfortably, ensuring your spine is straight and your feet are flat on the ground.
2. Rub your hands together briskly to generate warmth.
3. Gently cup your hands and place them over your eyes, ensuring no light seeps through. Your fingers should cross over the centre of your forehead, and your palms should allow your eyes to blink freely, not exerting pressure on the eyelids.
4. With your eyes closed beneath your palms, envision complete darkness and let your eyes bask in this tranquil space.

Deepening Relaxation

While the basic act of palming itself promotes relaxation, these advanced techniques can take it a notch higher:

1. **Breathing Synchronicity**: As you palm, focus on your breath. Take a deep breath in for a count of 4, hold for a count of 4, exhale for a count of 4, and wait for another count of 4 before inhaling again. This rhythmic breathing can amplify relaxation, allowing more oxygen to reach the eyes.

2. **Progressive Muscle Relaxation**: Before palming, take a few moments to tense and relax different muscle groups in your body. Start from your toes and move upwards, culminating in the muscles around your eyes. This helps in releasing residual tension.

3. **Environmental Enhancement**: Consider playing soft nature sounds or calming music in the background. The auditory stimulus can further deepen the relaxation experience during palming.

Visualizations and Palming

Visualization, a potent mental exercise, becomes more effective when paired with palming. The darkness and relaxation set a perfect stage for vivid mental imagery.

1. **Positive Memory Recall**: Within the darkness, recall a pleasant memory. Relive it, envisioning every detail - colours, sounds, sensations. The positive emotions drawn from this can counteract the stress that often contributes to vision problems.

2. **Journey to a Peaceful Place**: Imagine a serene place, perhaps a beach at sunset or a tranquil forest glade. Let your mind's eye observe every detail, from the distant horizons to the intricate patterns of leaves or grains of sand nearby.

3. **Dynamic Imagery**: Envision moving objects, like birds flying or leaves drifting in the wind. These moving images stimulate different parts of the visual system, further

enhancing the benefits of palming.

4. **Colour Meditation**: Visualize different colours one by one, letting each colour wash over your field of vision. Each hue can evoke unique emotions and responses, adding depth to the palming experience.

Consistency and Duration

While there's no strict rule on how long one should palm, for advanced practices, aim for at least 10-15 minutes to dive deep into relaxation and visualization. Consistency is crucial; daily palming sessions can significantly boost its therapeutic effects.

In Conclusion

Advanced palming techniques are more than just a vision exercise; they offer holistic benefits, rejuvenating the mind and body alongside the eyes. By integrating rhythmic breathing, muscle relaxation, and dynamic visualizations, one can elevate the simple act of palming into a profound meditative and restorative experience. Remember, vision is not just about clarity of sight but also clarity of mind. By harmonizing both, advanced palming offers a path to perfect sight without glasses.

CHAPTER 36: DYNAMIC FOCUSING TECHNIQUES

Vision is a dynamic process. From the moment we wake up to the second we drift into sleep, our eyes are constantly adjusting, focusing, and refocusing on various objects, both near and far. This innate ability is often taken for granted, but for some, the mechanism may be compromised, leading to visual discomfort or strain. This chapter sheds light on dynamic focusing techniques and provides insights into training the eyes to efficiently shift focus.

The Mechanics of Focusing

Before delving into the techniques, it's essential to understand the mechanics of focusing. The crystalline lens in our eye changes shape to focus light onto the retina. When we look at something up close, the lens becomes thicker. Conversely, when we gaze into the distance, the lens flattens. This adjustment is facilitated by the ciliary muscles, which contract or relax to change the lens's shape, enabling us to focus on objects at varying distances.

**Why is Dynamic Focusing Important? **

In our digital age, where screens dominate a significant portion of our waking hours, our eyes often remain fixed at one distance for extended periods. This static behavior can lead to eye strain, fatigue, and even a temporary condition called computer vision syndrome. Dynamic focusing exercises can alleviate these issues by promoting flexibility in the eye muscles and improving overall visual function.

Dynamic Focusing Techniques

1. **Pencil Push-ups**:
   - Begin by holding a pencil or any small object with writing on it at arm's length.
   - Focus on the text or a specific detail on the object.
   - Slowly bring the pencil closer to your nose while maintaining focus.
   - Stop once you notice double vision or can't keep the object in clear focus.
   - Return the pencil to its starting position and repeat the process 10-15 times.

2. **Distance Play**:
   - Sit by a window or in an open area with a clear view of distant objects.
   - Keep a book or any near object handy.
   - First, focus on the text or a detail on the near object for about 10 seconds.
   - Then, shift your gaze and focus on a distant object outside the window or in the open space for another 10 seconds.
   - Repeat this process for a few minutes, gradually increasing the time as your eyes become more adept at the exercise.

3. **Thumb Tracking**:
   - Extend one arm straight out, with your thumb pointing up.
   - Focus on your thumb.
   - Slowly move your thumb to the left, following it with your eyes without moving your head.
   - Bring your thumb back to the centre, then move it to the right, tracking it with your eyes.
   - Repeat this horizontal movement several times, then switch

to vertical movement — moving the thumb up and down.

4. **String Lights Technique**:
   - Tie small objects, like beads or paper pieces, at intervals on a long string.
   - Attach one end of the string to a wall and hold the other end on your nose, ensuring the string is taut.
   - Focus on each object sequentially, moving from the nearest to the farthest, then reversing the order.

Tips for Effective Practice:

1. **Posture**: Ensure you are seated comfortably with your back straight during these exercises. Proper alignment can prevent additional strain and enhance the effectiveness of the exercises.

2. **Blinking**: Remember to blink frequently to keep the eyes moistened. It helps reduce dryness and discomfort.

3. **Regular Breaks**: When working on a screen or doing any task that requires fixed focus for extended periods, practice the 20-20-20 rule: Every 20 minutes, take a 20-second break to gaze at something 20 feet away.

4. **Consistency**: Like any exercise regimen, the key to noticing improvement is consistency. Dedicate a few minutes every day to this dynamic focusing techniques.

In Conclusion

Dynamic focusing is an inherent skill that, unfortunately, many of us have let deteriorate due to modern lifestyle habits. However, with consistent practice of the techniques outlined above, one can not only combat the ill effects of prolonged screen time but also improve overall visual agility and health. By training the eyes to shift focus seamlessly from near too far and vice versa, we take a step closer to achieving perfect sight without glasses.

CHAPTER 37: DISTANCE VISION AND THE HORIZON GAZER

In our fast-paced, screen-dominant world, it's easy to forget the vastness that lies beyond our immediate surroundings. While our ancestors would regularly gaze across sprawling plains and vast landscapes, many of us are now confined to staring at devices mere inches from our faces. This shift has profound implications for our visual health and overall well-being. This chapter dives deep into the importance of distance vision and introduces the concept of the horizon gaze, emphasizing its significance in our journey to natural vision improvement.

The Importance of Looking Far

1. Natural Eye Relaxation: Our eyes are naturally attuned to viewing objects at a distance. When we gaze into the horizon or look far away, the eye muscles relax, and the lens inside the eye flattens. This state of relaxation reduces strain and tension, which are often caused by prolonged close-up tasks.

2. Improved Eye Function: Regularly practicing distance vision helps in maintaining the flexibility of the ciliary muscles, which control the shape of the eye's lens. This flexibility is essential for efficient switching between near and far vision.

3. Enhanced Depth Perception: Engaging with distant objects can improve depth perception, a crucial aspect of our visual system that helps us gauge distances and spatial relationships between objects.

4. Mental Well-being: There's a meditative quality to gazing into the horizon. The expansiveness can lead to feelings of calm and reduced mental stress, further promoting relaxation and clarity.

Exercises to Enhance Distance Vision

1. Horizon Gazing:
- Find a spot with a clear view of the horizon, like a hilltop, beach, or tall building.
- Sit or stand comfortably, relax your body, and take a few deep breaths.
- Softly gaze at the horizon line, trying not to blink excessively.
- Allow your eyes to scan the expanse from left to right and vice versa, noticing objects, colours, and movements.
- Practice this for 10-15 minutes daily, or as often as you can.

2. Far and Near Switch:
- Choose two objects: one close (within arm's reach) and one far away (as far off as possible).
- Start by focusing on the close object for about 10 seconds.
- Shift your gaze to the distant object, focusing on it for another 10 seconds.
- Repeat the process for a few minutes, gradually increasing the duration as you get comfortable.

3. Outdoor Reading:
- Grab a book or magazine and head outdoors.
- Find a location where you can intermittently read and then look up to gaze into the distance.
- Read a paragraph or page, then lift your head, focusing on a distant object or the horizon.

- Alternate between reading and distant gazing for about 20 minutes.

4. Landscape Exploration:
- Go on nature walks, hikes, or any outdoor activity that offers vast, open views.
- Make it a point to stop occasionally, soaking in the distant landscapes. Try to identify objects, shades, or movements.
- This exercise not only benefits your eyes but also connects you with nature, enhancing mental well-being.

Maintaining Distance Vision Health

1. **Limit Screen Time**: Make conscious efforts to break prolonged periods of screen use. Remember the 20-20-20 rule: every 20 minutes, take a 20-second break to view something 20 feet away.

2. **Engage in Outdoor Activities**: Activities like playing sports, gardening, or simply walking in a park can naturally encourage distance gazing.

3. **Mind Your Ergonomics**: Ensure your work or reading space is well-lit and ergonomically set up. Your screen or book should be at a comfortable distance, reducing the need for excessive close-up focus.

4. **Regular Eye Check-ups**: Visit an optometrist periodically to assess your vision and get recommendations tailored to your needs.

Conclusion

Distance vision, though seemingly simple, plays a pivotal role in our overall visual health. The horizon gaze, as an act of looking far and wide, is not just an exercise for the eyes, but also a reminder of the vastness and beauty that surrounds us. Embracing the horizon and practicing distance vision techniques can pave the way for improved eyesight and a deeper connection with the world around us.

CHAPTER 38: DEPTH PERCEPTION AND 3D VISION.

Depth perception, or the ability to perceive the world in three dimensions (3D) and judge the distance of objects, is a crucial aspect of our visual system. This perception is largely due to the binocular vision granted by our two forward-facing eyes. Together, they create a sense of depth, providing a fuller, richer visual experience. Let's delve into the intricacies of binocular vision and explore techniques that can refine our depth perception.

Binocular Vision: A Gift of Depth

Binocular vision arises from the slightly different views each of our eyes captures. When these separate images are processed by the brain, they converge into a single image with depth – a phenomenon called **stereopsis**. The slight difference between the images from each eye, known as **binocular disparity**, is the magic ingredient for our 3D vision.

The benefits of binocular vision include:

1. **Enhanced Field of View**: Two eyes positioned apart provide a wider view of our surroundings than a single eye would.
2. **Improved Visual Acuity**: By combining the images of both eyes, the brain can extract more details, enhancing our overall vision.

3. **3D Vision**: This allows us to judge distances, making activities like catching a ball, parking a car, or even threading a needle possible.

4. **Reduced Visual Blind Spots**: Each eye compensates for the other's blind spot.

However, for this system to work optimally, both eyes must work in harmony. If there's a misalignment or one eye is weaker, it can affect depth perception.

Techniques to Enhance Depth Perception

1. **Dot Stereograms**:
   - These are images with patterns of dots. When viewed with relaxed eyes, a hidden 3D image emerges.
   - Stare at the stereogram, letting your eyes lose focus slightly, almost like looking 'through' the image rather than 'at' it.
   - With practice, a 3D shape will appear, and this exercise can strengthen binocular vision and depth perception.

2. **Brock String Exercise**:
   - For this, you'll need a string around 10 feet long with three beads of different colours.
   - Attach one end of the string to a stationary object and hold the other end to your nose.
   - Space the beads a few inches apart along the string.
   - Focus on the closest bead. You should see two strings extending from the bead, forming an "X".
   - Shift focusses to the next bead. The "X" should now move to that bead. Continue with the third bead.
   - This exercise helps in training the eyes to work together and improve convergence, essential for depth perception.

3. **Pencil Push-Ups**:
   - Hold a pencil vertically with the eraser end up.
   - Extend your arm fully, then slowly move the pencil toward your nose, keeping your eyes focused on the eraser.
   - Stop when you see double or can't focus. Then, move the

pencil away and restart.
- This exercise strengthens the eye muscles and enhances convergence ability.

4. **Depth Jumping**:
- Choose two objects at different distances. For example, a book nearby and a door across the room.
- Quickly shift your focus from the near object to the far one, then back again.
- The rapid change in focus can improve depth perception and flexibility of the eye muscles.

5. **3D Video Games**:
- Some modern video games offer 3D experiences that can challenge and train depth perception. Engaging in these games, in moderation, can be both fun and beneficial for visual depth.

Maintaining Depth Perception Health

1. **Regular Eye Exams**: Regular check-ups can detect issues like lazy eye or misalignment early, both of which can affect depth perception.
2. **Active Lifestyle**: Engaging in sports, especially ball games, can naturally hone depth perception.
3. **Limit Screen Time**: Prolonged screen time can strain the eyes and affect their ability to switch focus between distances.
4. **Protect Your Eyes**: Ensure good lighting when reading or working and always protect your eyes from potential injuries.

Conclusion

Depth perception is a testament to the wonder that is our visual system. It allows us to navigate our world safely and efficiently. By understanding the mechanics of binocular vision and actively training our depth perception, we can ensure that we continue to experience the world in all its three-dimensional splendour.

CHAPTER 39: COLOUR PERCEPTION AND ITS IMPACT ON VISION

Colour paints our world with meaning, emotion, and beauty. Without the capacity to discern different colours, our experience of the world would be vastly different, even clinical. It's essential to understand the machinery behind colour perception, especially since it plays a significant role in the clarity and richness of our vision.

The Role of Cones in Colour Vision

In the human eye, two main types of photoreceptor cells are responsible for our ability to perceive light and colour: rods and cones. While rods are responsible for low-light vision, cones are the heroes behind our ability to perceive the vibrant colours of our environment.

1. **Structure and Function**: Cones are tapered cells situated in the retina, primarily in the macula and densely populated in the fovea centralis. This central region of the retina is where our visual acuity (sharpness) is the highest.

2. **Types of Cones**: There are three types of cone cells, each sensitive to different wavelengths of light:
   - **S-Cones**: Sensitive to short wavelengths, they perceive blue colours.
   - **M-Cones**: Sensitive to medium wavelengths, they capture

green colours.
   - **L-Cones**: Sensitive to long wavelengths, they detect red colours.

Our brain interprets the overlap and intensity of signals from these cones, enabling us to see a full spectrum of colours.

3. **Colour Blindness**: An anomaly in one or more types of cone cells can lead to colour vision deficiencies, commonly referred to as colour blindness. This can result in difficulty distinguishing between certain colours.

Exercises to Fine-Tune and Appreciate Colour Perception

1. **Colour Matching Game**:
   - Using coloured pencils or swatches, try to match the colours as closely as possible by memory.
   - This exercise trains your eyes to discern slight differences in shades and hues.

2. **Gradient Appreciation**:
   - Create or find a gradient sheet transitioning from one colour to another.
   - Spend time daily observing the subtle shifts in the gradient, focusing on areas where one colour morphs into the next.

3. **Nature Observation**:
   - Nature offers a vast array of colours, from the verdant greens of trees to the myriad colours of a sunset.
   - Take regular walks, pausing to observe and appreciate the richness of colours around you.

4. **Colour Meditation**:
   - Choose a colour that resonates with you on a given day.
   - Find a quiet spot and close your eyes, visualizing that colour filling your vision and mind.
   - This exercise not only boosts colour appreciation but also aids in relaxation.

5. **Colour Naming**:
   - Instead of generalizing colours as just red, blue, or green, try to name them more specifically, like crimson, turquoise, or lime. This exercise increases awareness and appreciation of the wide range of colours we can perceive.

6. **Afterimage Exercise**:
   - Stare at a brightly coloured object on a neutral background for about 30 seconds.
   - Quickly shift your gaze to a white wall or sheet of paper. You should see an afterimage in the complementary colour.
   - This phenomenon is a result of the cones' response to overstimulation, and it's a fun way to understand the workings of our colour vision.

7. **Art Appreciation**:
   - Engage in activities that use colours, such as painting, drawing, or even colouring books. This helps in honing your colour discernment skills and is therapeutic.

Conclusion

Colour perception is a marvellous capability that significantly enriches our life experiences. By understanding the role of cones and actively engaging in exercises to fine-tune our colour perception, we can further appreciate the vibrancy of our world. After all, in the words of artist Wassily Kandinsky, "Colour is a power which directly influences the soul." Embracing and nurturing our colour vision is not just about seeing but experiencing and feeling the world in its full chromatic splendour.

CHAPTER 40: EYE DOMINANCE: RECOGNIZING AND BALANCING

In many aspects of our lives, from writing to kicking a ball, we often favour one side of our body over the other. This natural inclination isn't just restricted to hands or feet; it extends to our eyes as well. Eye dominance, often referred to as 'ocular dominance,' is the tendency to prefer visual input from one eye over the other. Recognizing and understanding this dominance is crucial in many activities, from photography to sports like archery. But more than that, awareness of our eye dominance can be a tool for ensuring that both eyes are working in concert, promoting optimal visual health.

Identifying One's Dominant Eye

Before we can work on balancing our visual input, it's essential to identify which of our eyes is dominant. Here are some simple methods to determine your dominant eye:

1. **The Triangle Test**:
   - Extend your arms in front of you and create a small triangle between your thumbs and forefingers by touching them together.
   - Through this triangle, focus on a distant object, keeping both

eyes open.

- Close one eye at a time. The eye that keeps the object centred in the triangle, even when the other is closed, is your dominant eye.

2. **The Pointing Test**:

- Extend your arm and point at a distant object with your index finger.

- Close one eye at a time. The eye that has the finger pointing directly at the object, without any shift, is your dominant eye.

3. **The Reading Test**:

- Hold a book or any reading material at a comfortable distance.

- With both eyes open, focus on a specific word or letter.

- Close one eye at a time. The dominant eye will see the word or letter with minimal shift, while the other might see it off-position.

Activities to Ensure Both Eyes Work Harmoniously

While having a dominant eye is entirely normal, it's beneficial to ensure that both eyes are getting adequate stimulation and exercise. This harmony promotes depth perception, peripheral vision, and overall eye health. Here are some activities to encourage both eyes to work together:

1. **Alternate Eye Patching**:

- Spend some time each day wearing an eye patch over your dominant eye. This forces the non-dominant eye to take the lead, strengthening its visual acuity and muscles.

- Start with short intervals, like 5-10 minutes, and gradually increase as you become more comfortable.

2. **Mirror Drawing**:

- Using a mirror, try drawing a simple image or writing a sentence backward.

- This activity challenges your brain and eyes to coordinate in a new way, stimulating both eyes equally.

3. **Binocular Activities**:
   - Engage in activities that require the use of both eyes simultaneously, such as using binoculars, playing catch, or participating in 3D video games.
   - Such activities enhance binocular vision and depth perception.

4. **Switch Hands**:
   - If you're right-eyed dominant, try using your left hand for tasks like brushing teeth, eating, or writing and vice versa.
   - This cross-coordination can help balance the visual input from both eyes.

5. **Focus Shift Exercise**:
   - Hold a pen at arm's length and focus on its tip.
   - Slowly bring the pen closer to your nose, keeping focus on the tip.
   - Move it back out again.
   - This exercise ensures both eyes are working together to track the pen.

6. **Peripheral Vision Training**:
   - Place two small objects at eye level on either side of a room.
   - Standing in the middle, focus on a central point straight ahead.
   - Without moving your gaze from the centre, try to visually identify the objects in your peripheral vision. This exercise stimulates and balances the input from both eyes.

Conclusion

Awareness of our eye dominance offers more than just an interesting insight into our visual preference. It opens up avenues to strengthen, balance, and harmonize the input from both eyes, ensuring we maintain optimal vision and eye health throughout our lives. Like every other part of our body, our eyes too crave balance. By actively engaging in exercises that promote this equilibrium, we pave the way for clearer, healthier vision.

CHAPTER 41: IMPORTANCE OF REGULAR EYE EXAMINATIONS

Regular maintenance is essential for any system to function optimally, and our eyes are no exception. They are our windows to the world, playing a pivotal role in how we perceive, understand, and navigate our environment. Yet, we often take their well-being for granted. Regular eye examinations are crucial, not just to ensure we have the right vision correction but also to monitor for potential problems that can compromise our sight.

The Significance of Professional Eye Check-ups

1. **Early Detection of Eye Diseases**: Many eye diseases, like glaucoma or macular degeneration, manifest subtly in their early stages. Regular examinations can help in detecting these conditions early, allowing for timely intervention and potentially preserving vision.

2. **Ensuring Accurate Vision Correction**: Our eyes change over time. The prescription that worked for you a couple of years ago might not be suitable now. Regular check-ups ensure that any vision correction, whether glasses or contacts, is up-to-date and optimal.

3. **Detecting Other Health Issues**: Eyes can be the window to more than just the soul. Conditions like diabetes, high blood pressure, and even some tumours can be detected through comprehensive eye examinations.

4. **Assessing Functional Vision**: It's not just about clarity. How our eyes work together, depth perception, colour vision, and other aspects of functional vision are also assessed during a check-up.

5. **Eye Strain & Digital Eye Fatigue**: With the increasing screen time in our digital age, issues like digital eye strain have become more prevalent. Regular check-ups can help in providing guidance on managing and preventing such problems.

6. **Children's Vision**: Regular eye examinations are essential for children, ensuring that their vision develops appropriately. Undetected vision problems can lead to academic and developmental challenges.

What to Expect During an Eye Examination

1. **History Taking**: The optometrist will start by understanding your medical history, any vision problems you've been experiencing, and any family history of eye diseases.

2. **Vision Testing**: This will involve reading from an eye chart to determine the sharpness of your vision. Both distant and close-up vision will be tested.

3. **Pupil Dilation**: To get a better look at the internal structures of your eye, the optometrist might use drops to dilate your pupils. This provides a clearer view of the retina and optic nerve.

4. **Tonometry**: This test measures the pressure inside your eyes and is essential for detecting glaucoma.

5. **Peripheral Vision Testing**: This test will assess how well

you can see objects at the edge of your field of vision.

6. **Mobility Test**: This test evaluates the muscles controlling eye movement.

7. **Prescription for Corrective Lenses**: If you need glasses or contacts, the optometrist will determine the right prescription for you.

8. **Recommendations**: Based on your examination, the optometrist will provide guidance on eye care, potential treatments, or interventions if needed.

How Often to Visit an Optometrist

1. **Children (up to 18 years) **: An initial check-up in their first year, then at least once between the ages of 3 and 5, and annually after starting school.

2. **Adults (19 to 60 years) **: Every one to two years. However, if you have risk factors like diabetes, a family history of eye diseases, or currently wear glasses or contacts, annual check-ups are recommended.

3. **Seniors (61 years and above) **: Annually. As we age, the risk for eye diseases increases, making regular examinations even more vital.

4. **Contact Lens Wearers**: At least annually, as wearing contacts can increase the risk of eye infections.

Conclusion

Regular eye examinations are more than just a routine procedure; they're a cornerstone of maintaining optimal vision and eye health. They offer the advantage of early detection, prevention, and even the opportunity to enhance our visual experience. In our journey toward perfect sight without glasses, integrating the expertise of eye care professionals is invaluable. After all, the best care is a blend of natural practices and informed medical intervention.

CHAPTER 42: EXPLORING NATURAL AND HOLISTIC THERAPIES

Our eyes are more than just organs for sight; they are intricately connected to various systems within our body. As we journey through understanding vision and its improvement, it's crucial to explore the broader spectrum of holistic and alternative treatments. These therapies aim to treat the whole person, integrating the mind, body, and spirit. This chapter delves into acupuncture, reflexology, and other alternative treatments, assessing their potential benefits for vision health.

Acupuncture and Eye Health

Acupuncture, a cornerstone of traditional Chinese medicine, involves inserting fine needles into specific points on the body. The underlying philosophy is that our health depends on the balanced flow of "Qi" (life energy). Blockages or imbalances in this flow can lead to ailments.

Benefits for Vision Health:
1. **Glaucoma**: Some studies suggest that acupuncture can help reduce intraocular pressure and improve blood flow to the retina and optic nerve.
2. **Macular Degeneration**: Acupuncture may enhance retinal

function, helping in cases of age-related macular degeneration.
3. **Dry Eyes**: By improving the balance of Qi and enhancing blood flow, acupuncture can alleviate symptoms of dry eyes.

However, while some individuals find relief with acupuncture, it's essential to approach it as a complementary therapy and consult with ophthalmologists to understand its role in individual cases.

Reflexology for the Eyes

Reflexology is based on the principle that specific points on the feet, hands, and ears correspond to different body organs and systems. By massaging and applying pressure to these points, reflexologists believe that energy blockages can be released, promoting healing and balance.

Benefits for Vision Health:
1. **Eye Strain and Fatigue**: Reflexology can help relax the body, potentially reducing tension around the eyes.
2. **Headaches**: If your vision problems are accompanied by headaches, reflexology might offer relief by targeting points linked to head and eye tension.
3. **General Well-being**: As with many holistic treatments, the overall relaxation and balance achieved can indirectly support eye health.

Other Alternative Treatments

1. **Ayurveda**: This ancient Indian system of medicine suggests that imbalances in the body's three "doshas" can lead to health problems, including eye issues. Specific diets, herbal treatments, and practices like "netra basti" (a treatment involving warm ghee on the eyes) are prescribed based on one's constitution and imbalances.

2. **Bates Method**: Developed by Dr. William H. Bates in the early 20th century, this method focuses on relaxing the eye muscles, visual training, and creating good visual habits to

improve eyesight naturally.

3. **Herbal Remedies**: Various herbs like bilberry, ginkgo biloba, and goji berries have been touted for their potential benefits for eye health, primarily due to their antioxidant properties.

4. **Nutrition Therapy**: The importance of a balanced diet rich in vitamins (like vitamin A and E) and minerals (like zinc) cannot be understated. Omega-3 fatty acids, found in fish and flaxseeds, have also been linked to better eye health.

Benefits for Vision Health:
1. **Prevention of Diseases**: Many alternative treatments focus on prevention, ensuring that the eyes remain healthy.
2. **Holistic Improvement**: By focusing on the body as a whole, these therapies can address underlying issues that indirectly impact vision.

Conclusion

When exploring natural and holistic therapies, it's essential to approach them with an open yet discerning mind. While many individuals have found relief and improvement in their vision through these methods, they are best used in conjunction with, and not as a replacement for, conventional medical advice and treatments.

As with all health decisions, individual research, consulting with experts, and listening to one's body are paramount. The goal is to create a personalized, integrative approach to vision health, drawing from the best of both conventional and alternative worlds. In our quest for perfect sight without glasses, the more tools we have in our toolkit, the better equipped we are to achieve our vision goals.

CHAPTER 43: LIFESTYLE FACTORS AFFECTING VISION

In our pursuit of perfect sight without glasses, it's vital to recognize the profound impact our lifestyle choices have on our vision health. From the foods we consume to the air we breathe, every choice leaves an imprint on our eyes. This chapter delves into the more prominent lifestyle factors, particularly smoking, alcohol, and other habits, and highlights positive changes one can adopt to bolster eye health.

The Smoky Haze: Impact of Smoking on Eyesight

It's common knowledge that smoking is detrimental to the lungs and heart, but its harmful effects on our eyes are often overlooked.

Detrimental Effects:
1. **Cataracts**: Smoking doubles the chance of forming cataracts, which cloud the eye's lens, leading to blurred vision.
2. **Macular Degeneration**: This age-related condition affects the central part of the retina, which is responsible for sharp vision. Smokers are at a higher risk.
3. **Uveitis**: Smoking increases the risk of this severe eye condition, which can lead to complete blindness.
4. **Dry Eyes**: The smoke and chemicals in cigarettes aggravate the eye, leading to dryness and discomfort.

Alcohol's Blur: Vision Impairment through Excessive Drinking

While moderate alcohol consumption might have some health benefits, excessive drinking can negatively impact vision.

Effects on Vision:
1. **Macular Degeneration**: Chronic alcohol consumption can increase the risk of developing age-related macular degeneration.
2. **Cataracts**: High alcohol intake has been linked to an increased chance of cataract formation.
3. **Vision Changes**: Alcohol can affect the way the eyes' function, leading to blurred or double vision, and decreased peripheral vision.
4. **Optic Neuropathy**: Excessive drinking can lead to this condition, where vision loss is due to damage to the optic nerve.

Other Lifestyle Habits and Their Impacts

1. **Diet**: A poor diet lacking essential vitamins and minerals can weaken vision. Nutrients like vitamin C, E, zinc, and carotenoids are crucial for maintaining healthy eyesight.
2. **Lack of Exercise**: Physical inactivity can increase the risk of conditions like diabetes, which in turn can lead to eye problems like diabetic retinopathy.
3. **Exposure to Sun**: Extended exposure to the sun's ultraviolet rays without protection can damage the eyes and increase the risk of cataracts and macular degeneration.
4. **Digital Strain**: Prolonged screen time without breaks can cause digital eye strain, leading to blurred vision, dry eyes, and headaches.

Positive Lifestyle Changes for Eye Health

1. **Quit Smoking**: Ceasing smoking can reduce the risk of several eye conditions. It's never too late to quit, and the eyes can benefit from improved circulation and reduced exposure to

toxins.

2. **Limit Alcohol**: Drinking in moderation, if at all, can prevent the adverse effects of alcohol on the eyes.

3. **Balanced Diet**: Incorporate a diet rich in colorful fruits and vegetables. Omega-3 fatty acids, found in fish, can also promote healthy vision.

4. **Regular Exercise**: Engaging in physical activity can reduce the risk of systemic conditions that threaten vision.

5. **Protect Your Eyes**: Always wear sunglasses with UV protection when outdoors. If you're working in front of screens, make sure to take regular breaks using the 20-20-20 rule.

6. **Stay Hydrated**: Drinking sufficient water supports natural tear production, helping prevent dry eyes.

Conclusion

Our eyes are a reflection of our overall health, and the lifestyle choices we make play a pivotal role in determining their well-being. Adopting positive habits while shedding harmful ones can pave the way for clearer, healthier vision. After all, the journey towards perfect sight without glasses is not just about eye exercises and relaxation techniques; it's also about nurturing our bodies and making choices that sustain and enhance our visual health.

CHAPTER 44: PRESERVING VISION AS WE AGE

The aging process is a natural part of life, and just as our skin, hair, and joints undergo changes over time, so too do our eyes. However, growing older doesn't necessarily mean having to accept poor vision. Understanding the age-related changes in vision and adopting proactive strategies can assist us in maintaining and even enhancing our eyesight during our golden years.

Natural Age-related Changes in Vision

As we age, several changes occur in our eyes:

1. **Presbyopia**: Around the age of 40, many people start to experience difficulty in focusing on close objects. This condition, known as presbyopia, results from the lens of the eye becoming less flexible over time.

2. **Reduced Pupil Size**: The pupil shrinks and becomes less responsive to changes in ambient lighting, making older individuals more sensitive to glare and requiring more time to adjust to different lighting conditions.

3. **Decreased Colour Vision**: The clear lens inside our eye can discolour over time, leading to a reduced sensitivity to variations in colour.

4. **Vitreous Detachment**: The gel-like substance (vitreous) inside the eyes can begin to liquefy and potentially pull away from the retina. While often harmless, it can sometimes lead to more serious conditions.

5. **Common Eye Diseases**: Age increases the risk of several eye diseases, including cataracts, glaucoma, and age-related macular degeneration.

Strategies to Maintain and Enhance Vision in Later Years

Though age-related changes in vision are natural, they don't have to limit our quality of life. By adopting specific strategies, we can preserve, and in some cases, improve our eyesight as we age:

1. **Regular Eye Exams**: This cannot be emphasized enough. Regular visits to the optometrist or ophthalmologist can detect early signs of eye diseases, many of which are treatable if caught early.

2. **Nutritious Diet**: Consuming a diet rich in antioxidants, vitamins, and minerals can support eye health. Leafy greens, berries, oily fish, nuts, and seeds are all excellent choices.

3. **Adequate Lighting**: With age, our eyes require lighter to see clearly. Ensure that your home is well-lit, especially in areas where you read or perform detailed tasks.

4. **Limit UV Exposure**: Always wear sunglasses with UVA and UVB protection when outdoors. Extended exposure to the sun's ultraviolet rays can worsen cataracts and increase the risk of macular degeneration.

5. **Stay Active**: Physical activity promotes good circulation, which is beneficial for eye health. Simple activities like walking can make a significant difference.

6. **Limit Screen Time**: Prolonged exposure to digital screens

can strain the eyes. If you spend a lot of time on computers or mobile devices, remember to take frequent breaks.

7. **Protective Eyewear**: When engaging in activities that could pose a risk to your eyes, like gardening, woodworking, or playing certain sports, always wear protective glasses.

8. **Manage Chronic Conditions**: Diabetes, high blood pressure, and other systemic conditions can adversely affect vision. Regular check-ups and proper management can prevent related eye complications.

9. **Stay Hydrated**: Drink ample water to support natural tear production, which can decline with age, leading to dry eyes.

10. **Limit Alcohol and Quit Smoking**: Both excessive drinking and smoking can exacerbate age-related eye problems.

11. **Engage in Eye Exercises**: Incorporate exercises like palming, zooming, and figure-of-eight into your routine. These exercises can improve focus, enhance peripheral vision, and reduce strain.

12. **Stay Mentally Active**: Engaging in puzzles, reading, or learning new skills can keep the mind and eyes sharp.

Conclusion

Aging might be inevitable, but compromised vision doesn't have to be a given. With proactive care, awareness, and a commitment to overall well-being, we can ensure that our eyes remain one of our most cherished assets, allowing us to explore, learn, and experience the beauty of the world around us, no matter our age. Remember, preserving our sight as we age begins with understanding the changes our eyes undergo and taking deliberate steps to support and enhance our vision throughout our lifetime.

CHAPTER 45: CORRECTING LAZY EYE (AMBLYOPIA) NATURALLY

Amblyopia, commonly known as "lazy eye," is a vision disorder that arises when one eye doesn't develop normal sight. Typically manifesting in early childhood, it's not merely a cosmetic issue; the term "lazy" can be misleading. If left untreated, it can result in permanent vision impairment. But how can one address it naturally? Here's a deep dive into understanding this condition and some holistic approaches to its improvement.

Understanding the Causes and Symptoms of Amblyopia

Amblyopia occurs when the brain and one eye don't work cohesively, leading the brain to favour the other eye. Over time, the disregarded eye tends to wander inwards or outwards, leading to the common term "lazy eye."

There are three primary causes:

1. **Strabismic Amblyopia**: This is the result of misaligned eyes, where one eye might turn in, out, up, or down.

2. **Refractive Amblyopia**: Here, one eye has a significantly different prescription than the other. One eye may be more near-sighted, farsighted, or have more astigmatism.

3. **Deprivation Amblyopia**: This is caused by an obstruction to vision, such as cataract, preventing clear vision in that eye.

Symptoms include:

- Eyes that wander inwards or outwards.
- Poor depth perception.
- Squinting or shutting an eye.
- Head tilting.
- Noticeable visual impairment in one eye.

Exercises and Techniques to Address and Improve Amblyopia

Holistic approaches focus on strengthening the weaker eye, enhancing brain-eye coordination, and ensuring both eyes work in harmony. Here are some natural techniques:

1. **Patch Therapy**: This is the most traditional method. By placing a patch over the stronger eye, the weaker eye is forced to work harder, strengthening its connection to the brain. Initially, tasks can be simple like colouring or reading, gradually moving to more complex activities.

2. **Near and Far Focus**: Hold a small object, like a pen, at arm's length and focus on it. Slowly move it closer until it's about six inches from your nose. Then move it away again. Repeat this exercise for a few minutes daily, ensuring the "lazy eye" is doing the majority of the work.

3. **Brock String**: This involves a string with three beads of different colours. The goal is to focus on each bead, promoting convergence and enhancing depth perception.

4. **Pendulum Exercise**: Watch a pendulum or a swinging necklace, ensuring the lazy eye is leading in the tracking, strengthening eye muscles and coordination.

5. **Computer Programs and Apps**: Today, several computerized training programs are designed to improve

amblyopia. They involve games and tasks that challenge both eyes to work together.

6. **Contrast Sensitivity Training**: This involves identifying and distinguishing various shades of the same colour. There are charts and apps designed for this purpose.

7. **Balancing Exercises**: Standing on one leg, tossing a ball, or using a balance board can help improve visual input and enhance eye-brain coordination.

8. **Diet and Nutrition**: Omega-3 fatty acids, found in fish, flaxseeds, and walnuts, can support vision development. Lutein and zeaxanthin, found in green leafy vegetables, can also be beneficial.

It's essential to approach amblyopia holistically, combining exercises with regular check-ups and professional guidance. Starting early provides the best chance for improvement, but even adults with amblyopia can benefit from these natural techniques.

Remember, every individual's experience with amblyopia is unique. What works for one person might not work for another. It's about finding the right combination of exercises and being consistent with them. With patience, persistence, and the right approach, improvement is entirely possible.

CHAPTER 46: CHILDREN'S VISION: EARLY CARE AND HABITS

From the first moment a baby locks eyes with its parent, the journey of visual development commences. Vision is intrinsic to how children comprehend the world around them. From reading to writing, from playing catch to drawing, clear sight is pivotal. It's essential, then, to ensure that our children's eyes are given the best care from the outset, and habits developed early can have lifelong benefits.

Recognizing Vision Problems in Children

Children might not always vocalize or even recognize vision issues since they might assume that everyone sees the way they do. Hence, it's crucial for parents and caregivers to be vigilant about any signs of vision problems. Here are some indicators:

1. **Squinting or Closing One Eye**: If a child frequently squints or closes one eye, especially when focusing on distant objects or reading, it might be an indication of a refractive error.

2. **Frequent Eye Rubbing**: While occasional rubbing is normal, if a child does it persistently, it may signal eye fatigue or discomfort.

3. **Sitting Too Close to Screens**: Children preferring to sit unusually close to the television or holding devices very near might be compensating for near-sightedness.

4. **Avoiding Reading or Other Visual Tasks**: A child avoiding books or visual tasks may be finding it hard to focus, indicating potential vision problems.

5. **Tilting Head or Unusual Postures**: Adopting strange postures or tilting the head can be a child's instinctual way of adjusting to vision discrepancies between the eyes.

6. **Frequent Headaches**: Repeated headaches, especially after visual tasks, can be a sign of eye strain.

7. **Difficulty Following Moving Objects**: If a child struggles to track or follow moving objects, it could signify issues with eye muscle control.

Regular eye examinations are essential, as many vision problems can be corrected if diagnosed early.

Instilling Good Vision Habits from a Young Age

Children's eyes are malleable and responsive to their environment. The habits they develop early on can set the foundation for a lifetime of good vision.

1. **Regular Breaks**: Children, especially in this digital age, spend ample time in front of screens. Ensure they take breaks every 20 minutes, looking 20 feet away for 20 seconds – the 20-20-20 rule.

2. **Proper Lighting**: Make sure their reading or study area is well-lit, ideally with natural light, to reduce eye strain.

3. **Limit Screen Time**: While it's challenging in today's world, it's crucial to set limits on how long children can use devices. Encourage outdoor play, which not only benefits their vision but their overall health.

4. **Eye Exercises**: Just like any muscles, the eyes benefit from workouts. Teach children simple exercises like tracing imaginary figures with their eyes or the near-far focus technique.

5. **Nutrition**: A balanced diet rich in omega-3s, vitamin C, E, and zinc can boost eye health. Foods like fish, nuts, citrus fruits, green leafy vegetables, and eggs are all excellent choices.

6. **Protective Wear**: If your child is involved in sports or activities that might pose a risk to their eyes, ensure they wear protective eyewear.

7. **Book Position**: Teach children to hold their books or devices at about the distance of their elbow to their eyes, which is a comfortable distance for reading.

8. **Promote Blinking**: Remind children to blink frequently, especially when they're engrossed in screens. Blinking moistens the eyes, reducing the risk of dryness and irritation.

9. **Early Eye Exams**: Children should have their first comprehensive eye exam at six months, then at age three, and again before they start school. Regular check-ups can catch and correct potential issues early on.

In conclusion, vision is a treasured gift, and childhood is the ideal time to lay the foundation for a lifetime of clear sight. Recognizing issues early and instilling the right habits can make a world of difference. As with all things concerning our children, it's about guidance, consistency, and providing the best tools and habits for a bright, visually rich future.

CHAPTER 47: DEALING WITH COMMON EYE AILMENTS

Our eyes, though intricate and resilient, are not immune to occasional hiccups. Common eye ailments can range from the mildly irritating to those demanding more attention. Understanding these conditions and knowing how to manage them can provide comfort and prevent further complications.

Overview of Common Eye Ailments

1. **Dry Eyes**: This condition occurs when your tears aren't able to provide adequate lubrication. Symptoms include a stinging or burning sensation, stringy mucus in or around the eyes, increased eye irritation from wind or smoke, sensitivity to light, and difficulty wearing contact lenses.

2. **Pink Eye (Conjunctivitis)**: This is an inflammation or infection of the transparent membrane that lines your eyelid and covers the white part of your eyeball. Symptoms include redness, itchiness, a gritty feeling, discharge that forms a crust, and tearing.

3. **Styes**: A stye is a painful, red lump on the edge of your eyelid, near the base of the eyelashes. It often looks like a pimple and can be filled with pus.

Natural Remedies and Preventive Care

1. **Dry Eyes**:
   - *Warm Compress*: A warm, damp cloth held over your eyes can help stimulate tear production and alleviate dryness.
   - *Blink Regularly*: Especially when reading or staring at a computer screen for long periods, remember to blink often to moisten your eyes.
   - *Stay Hydrated*: Drinking plenty of water can help flush out salt from the body and properly hydrate your eyes, reducing the symptoms of dryness.
   - *Omega-3s*: Incorporating omega-3 fatty acids in your diet (from foods like flaxseeds, walnuts, and fish) can help improve the oil quality in tears, reducing dry eye symptoms.

2. **Pink Eye (Conjunctivitis)**:
   - *Cool Compress*: For allergic conjunctivitis, a cool compress can help ease the itchiness and inflammation.
   - *Avoid Touching*: It's crucial not to touch the affected eye and to wash hands regularly. Conjunctivitis can be contagious, so maintaining hygiene is essential.
   - *Honey*: Some believe diluted honey can offer relief due to its antibacterial properties. However, always consult with an eye specialist before trying home remedies.
   - *Green Tea*: Using a cold, damp green tea bag on the infected eye can provide relief due to its anti-inflammatory properties.

3. **Styes**:
   - *Warm Compress*: Applying a warm compress several times daily can help the stye come to a head and drain on its own.
   - *Clean the Eyelid*: Using baby shampoo diluted with warm water and cleaning your eyelids can help prevent further infections.
   - *Avoid Popping*: Do not attempt to squeeze or pop a stye, as this can spread the infection.
   - *Turmeric*: This has natural anti-inflammatory and antibacterial properties. Drinking turmeric milk or applying a paste (after consulting with an expert) may aid recovery.

General Preventive Care for Eye Health:

- **Regular Cleaning**: Wash your hands regularly and avoid touching your eyes. This simple habit can prevent a variety of eye ailments.

- **Maintain Hygiene with Contact Lenses**: If you wear contacts, ensure you clean them regularly, avoid wearing them longer than recommended, and always handle with clean hands.

- **Stay Hydrated**: A well-hydrated body ensures well-lubricated eyes.

- **Balanced Diet**: Nutrients like omega-3 fatty acids, lutein, zinc, and vitamins C and E can help ward off age-related vision problems. Include green leafy veggies, fish, eggs, nuts, beans, and other protein sources in your diet.

- **Wear Sunglasses**: Shield your eyes from the harmful UV rays of the sun. Choose sunglasses that block 99% to 100% of both UVA and UVB rays.

- **Reduce Screen Time**: Limit the amount of time spent in front of screens and adopt the 20-20-20 rule to reduce eye strain.

- **Annual Eye Exams**: Regular eye check-ups can pre-empt many eye ailments and ensure that any issues are dealt with promptly.

In conclusion, while common eye ailments can be a nuisance, understanding their nature and knowing how to address them naturally can provide relief. However, always consult with a healthcare professional before starting any natural remedies, especially when it concerns the eyes. The adage remains true: prevention is better than cure. Maintain good eye hygiene, adopt a balanced lifestyle, and prioritize your eye health daily.

CHAPTER 48: NATURAL VISION IMPROVEMENT SUCCESS STORIES

Embarking on a journey toward natural vision improvement can be met with scepticism and uncertainty. However, numerous individuals have already blazed this trail, with noteworthy results that bolster the promise of these holistic approaches. This chapter presents a collection of their inspiring stories, shedding light on the potential of natural methods.

1. Jenna's Journey from Glasses to Clarity

Jenna had been wearing glasses since she was six years old. As she entered her thirties, she grew frustrated with the increasing dependency on her spectacles. She recalls, "I felt chained. Whether I was reading, driving, or simply looking at the faces of my children, I was lost without my glasses."

After coming across a book on natural vision improvement, Jenna decided to incorporate eye exercises into her daily routine. She practiced palming, sunning, and the 20-20-20 rule diligently. Six months into her journey, she noticed that her eyes felt less strained, and she began forgetting her glasses at home without much inconvenience. "It was liberating," Jenna shares. "It felt as if my eyes were gradually waking up from a long slumber." Today, Jenna only uses her glasses for night-time driving and has reduced her prescription by half.

2. Raj's Triumph Over Digital Eye Strain

An IT professional, Raj spent over 12 hours daily in front of screens. He began experiencing severe headaches, blurry vision, and persistent eye fatigue. "My work was suffering," Raj admits. "I tried anti-glare glasses, but they only provided temporary relief."

Introduced to dynamic focusing techniques by a friend, Raj started taking regular screen breaks, shifting his focus from his monitor to distant objects every 20 minutes. He also practiced eye massages and used warm compresses in the evenings. Within weeks, Raj's symptoms began to diminish. "Not only has my eye strain reduced significantly," Raj beams, "but my overall productivity and mood have improved too."

3. Maria's Conquest of Astigmatism

Maria had astigmatism, a refractive error caused by an irregularly shaped cornea. Rather than opt for corrective surgery or rely solely on lenses, she decided to explore natural ways to manage her condition.

She began with a dedicated routine of Bates exercises, including swinging and visualizing techniques. Maria also practiced gazing exercises, wherein she'd focus on objects at various distances without squinting or straining. "It was tough initially," Maria confesses. "But I was patient and persistent." Over time, Maria experienced a noticeable improvement in her vision clarity. While her astigmatism wasn't completely cured, her dependency on corrective lenses reduced remarkably. "The world looks different when you can see it without a crutch," she reflects.

4. Alex's Battle with Amblyopia

Diagnosed with amblyopia or 'lazy eye' as a child, Alex wore an eye patch to help correct the imbalance between his eyes. "Kids at school used to tease me," Alex recalls. As an adult, while the amblyopia was less pronounced, Alex felt his vision could be better.

After researching holistic vision techniques, he began incorporating patching with focused eye exercises, alternating between his eyes to promote balance. He also engaged in activities that required depth perception and coordination, like juggling. Today, Alex's eyes work more harmoniously than ever. "It's a journey, but the progress is undeniable," he states.

Insights and Inspirations

These stories underscore a common theme: the incredible adaptability and resilience of our eyes. While results vary, the potential for improvement through dedication, patience, and consistent practice is evident.

For readers contemplating their journey toward natural vision improvement, these stories serve as beacons of hope and motivation. While each individual's experience is unique, the shared essence of triumph over adversity offers encouragement.

It's essential to remember that natural vision improvement doesn't promise miraculous cures. Instead, it offers a holistic approach to understanding, nurturing, and harnessing the potential within our eyes. As these narratives suggest, with commitment and belief, we can reframe our vision stories, shaping them into tales of empowerment and success.

CHAPTER 49: KEEPING A VISION JOURNAL

Journeying towards better eyesight through natural methods is akin to setting out on a path of self-discovery. Every step, every realization, and every subtle change can be a valuable lesson. Capturing these moments can be profoundly beneficial, and this is where the idea of a vision journal comes into play.

Understanding the Concept of a Vision Journal

A vision journal is not merely a record of how well you see but an in-depth account of your experiences, feelings, challenges, and triumphs as you work towards improving your eyesight. It encapsulates both the objective and the subjective, providing a comprehensive look into your journey.

Benefits of Tracking One's Progress

1. **Reflection and Awareness**: A journal serves as a mirror, reflecting your experiences, allowing you to discern patterns, habits, and triggers that affect your vision. By regularly penning down your observations, you become more attuned to your body's signals and responses.

2. **Motivation**: On days when you feel disheartened, revisiting earlier entries and recognizing how far you've come can serve as a powerful motivator. Every small victory documented can reignite your determination.

3. **Personal Accountability**: Regularly updating your journal

encourages a sense of responsibility towards your vision-improvement goals.

4. **Informed Decision Making**: Should you wish to modify your regimen or introduce new techniques, your journal entries provide valuable data, helping you make informed choices.

Tips for Maintaining a Personal Vision Diary

1. **Consistency is Key**: Choose a fixed time daily, perhaps every evening, to reflect on the day and document your experiences. It's the habit of writing, more than the length of the entry, that matters.

2. **Structure Your Entries**: While some prefer a free-flowing format, others might benefit from a structured approach. Consider sections like:
   - *Date and Time*: To keep track of your progress.
   - *Exercises Practiced*: Detail the techniques you tried and for how long.
   - *Observations*: Note any immediate effects, difficulties, or breakthroughs.
   - *General Health and Mood*: Your overall well-being can significantly influence your vision.
   - *Special Notes*: Any deviations from the routine, like missing an exercise, trying a new one, or experiencing particular stressors.

3. **Include Visual Tests**: Every once in a while, test your vision in a consistent setting—like reading a specific chart or recognizing distant objects—and note your observations.

4. **Embrace Honesty**: Your journal is a personal space. Be honest about your feelings, frustrations, and achievements. It's essential to acknowledge both challenges and progress.

5. **Review Regularly**: Set aside time, perhaps monthly, to review your entries. This not only helps gauge your progress but can also offer insights into areas that need more focus.

6. **Personalize Your Journal**: Make it a space you love. Use colours, sketches, or stickers. The more invested you are in the journal, the more likely you are to use it consistently.

7. **Stay Positive**: While it's vital to note down challenges, try to maintain a positive tone. Celebrate small victories and be compassionate towards yourself on tougher days.

Reviewing and Drawing Insights

As months pass, your vision journal will grow rich with data. Periodic reviews will highlight:
- Patterns in mood and well-being affecting your vision.
- Specific exercises that yield better results for you.
- Times when you faced challenges, and how you overcame them.

Drawing insights from these can help refine your approach, making your journey more effective and personalized.

In Conclusion

A vision journal goes beyond mere record-keeping; it's a companion on your journey towards better eyesight. As you navigate the ups and downs of natural vision improvement, this journal will stand testament to your commitment, progress, and the profound connection between mind, body, and vision. Embrace it, for in its pages lie the chronicles of your unique path to clearer sight.

Part V: Overcoming Challenges

CHAPTER 50: DEALING WITH DOUBTS AND SCEPTICISM

Embracing the journey of natural vision improvement is both exciting and challenging. One of the most significant challenges many faces is not the regimen itself, but the cloud of doubt and scepticism that might surround such an unconventional approach. Scepticism can emerge from within oneself, or it can be the result of external voices — friends, family, or even medical professionals who might not fully endorse these methods.

Understanding the Roots of Scepticism

Before diving into strategies to combat scepticism, it's crucial to understand its origins. Historically, conventional medicine has been the primary route for most ailments, including vision problems. Anything that diverges from this norm can, understandably, raise eyebrows. Additionally, the plethora of quick-fix scams in the world of health and wellness further fuels scepticism around legitimate natural techniques.

1. Internal Doubt

* **Impatience**: Natural vision improvement is a gradual process. It's easy to get impatient and doubt the efficacy when immediate results aren't visible.
* **Comparison with Others**: Every individual's journey is

unique. Comparing one's progress with someone else's can lead to feelings of inadequacy and doubt.

2. External Scepticism

* **Lack of Awareness**: Many are unfamiliar with natural vision improvement techniques, leading to scepticism.
* **Contradictory Views**: You might come across professionals or articles that don't support these methods, leading to external doubt.

Staying Committed Amidst the Scepticism

1. **Educate Yourself**: The more you know about natural vision improvement techniques, the better equipped you are to deal with scepticism. Dive deep into the science and success stories. Knowledge is not just power; it's confidence.

2. **Find a Supportive Community**: There are numerous forums, groups, and communities that advocate natural vision improvement. Being a part of such a community can provide much-needed encouragement. Sharing experiences, challenges, and successes with like-minded individuals can be immensely uplifting.

3. **Maintain a Vision Journal**: As discussed in the previous chapter, a vision journal can be a testament to your progress. On days filled with doubt, revisiting your journal can remind you of how far you've come.

4. **Respectful Dialogue with Sceptics**: When faced with external scepticism, engage in open dialogue. Sharing your experiences, reasons, and the science behind your choices might not convert sceptics but can foster understanding.

5. **Trust the Process**: Understand that natural vision improvement is not an overnight miracle. It's a journey, with its ups and downs. Trusting the process means having faith even when the results are not immediate.

6. **Seek Professional Guidance**: While many optometrists might lean towards conventional methods, there are professionals who endorse and support natural techniques. Seeking advice from them can provide validation and reassurance.

7. **Reframe Your Mindset**: Instead of viewing natural vision improvement as a strict regimen with an end goal, consider it a lifestyle choice, akin to opting for a balanced diet or regular exercise. This shift in perspective can reduce performance pressure and help you enjoy the journey.

8. **Limit Negative Influences**: While it's essential to remain open-minded, continuously exposing oneself to negative or contradictory views can be draining. Limit such exposures and focus on what resonates with you.

9. **Celebrate Small Wins**: Every bit of progress, no matter how minor it might seem, is a step forward. Celebrate these moments. They serve as tangible evidence against scepticism.

10. **Revisit Your 'Why'**: On particularly challenging days, revisit the reasons why you started this journey. Was it to avoid glasses? To lead a healthier life? To challenge the conventional? Reconnecting with your motivations can reignite passion and commitment.

Conclusion

Embarking on a journey of natural vision improvement is a personal choice, one that might not always align with popular opinion. Doubts and scepticism are natural companions on this journey. However, with the right tools, mindset, and support, they can be overcome. Your vision's health and clarity are worth every challenge, every sceptic's comment, and every momentary doubt. Stay committed, trust the process, and let your experiences guide you. Remember, the clearest vision is not just about seeing the world but understanding oneself.

CHAPTER 51: TROUBLESHOOTING PLATEAUS

In the journey towards natural vision improvement, much like any endeavour that requires commitment and effort, there might come a time when progress seems to halt. These plateaus can be frustrating, leading many to question the effectiveness of their efforts or even consider giving up. This chapter is dedicated to understanding these plateaus and offering guidance on how to navigate them.

Understanding Plateaus in Vision Improvement

A plateau in vision improvement is characterized by a period where no noticeable progress is made despite consistent efforts. Several reasons can contribute to this stalling:

1. **The Body's Natural Adaptation**: Over time, our bodies adapt to the exercises and techniques we employ. What once posed a challenge and induced change might no longer have the same effect.

2. **Overexertion**: Paradoxically, trying too hard or over-practicing can sometimes hinder progress. Overstraining the eyes might lead to fatigue, which can counteract improvement efforts.

3. **Incomplete Techniques**: While practicing vision exercises, it's possible to overlook certain aspects or not perform them in

their entirety.

4. **External Factors**: Stress, lack of sleep, poor diet, and other external factors can significantly impact vision improvement.

Navigating Through Plateaus

1. **Re-Evaluate Your Techniques**: Go back to the basics. Ensure that you're practicing the exercises correctly. Sometimes, small tweaks in technique can yield significant results.

2. **Introduce Variability**: If you've been doing the same set of exercises for a long time, consider mixing them up. The eyes, like any other part of our body, benefit from varied stimulation.

3. **Prioritize Rest**: Ensure that you're giving your eyes adequate rest. Incorporate regular breaks, especially if you have screen-intensive tasks. Revisit the chapter on 'The Role of Sleep in Vision Health' to ensure you're getting quality rest.

4. **Address External Factors**: Analyze other aspects of your life that might be impacting your vision. Are you managing stress effectively? Are your diet rich in nutrients beneficial for eye health? Addressing these factors can sometimes jumpstart progress.

5. **Stay Committed**: A plateau, while challenging, is not a dead end. Stay committed to the journey. The body has its rhythms of progress, and patience is key.

6. **Seek Expert Advice**: If you've tried multiple strategies and still find yourself at a standstill, consider consulting with a professional familiar with natural vision improvement. They might offer insights or modifications that you hadn't considered.

7. **Group Support**: Joining a group or community of individuals on a similar journey can be helpful. Sharing experiences and tips can offer fresh perspectives. Sometimes, just knowing that others have faced and overcome similar

challenges can be immensely motivating.

8. **Celebrate the Journey**: Instead of focusing solely on the end goal, celebrate the journey. Appreciate the improvements you've made thus far, even if they seem minor.

9. **Mental Imagery and Relaxation**: Sometimes, mental blocks can contribute to physical plateaus. Practices like visualization and relaxation can help break these barriers. Techniques like advanced palming, which incorporates deep relaxation and visualization, can be particularly beneficial during plateaus.

10. **Reassess Goals**: It might be a good time to revisit and reassess your vision goals. Perhaps they need to be more specific, or maybe they need to be set in smaller, more achievable increments.

Conclusion

Experiencing a plateau can be disheartening, but it's a natural part of any growth journey. It's crucial to approach plateaus with a mindset of curiosity rather than frustration. Often, they serve as opportunities to refine techniques, introduce variability, and deepen understanding. With persistence, commitment, and the right strategies, plateaus can be surmounted, paving the way for continued progress and clearer vision. Remember, every challenge faced and overcome is a testament to your dedication and a step closer to perfect sight without glasses.

CHAPTER 52: THE ROLE OF EMOTIONAL WELL-BEING IN VISION HEALTH

Emotional well-being is intrinsically linked to our overall health, and our eyes are no exception. The eyes, often hailed as the windows to the soul, have more to reveal than we might realize at first glance. Understanding the profound connection between our emotional states and vision is vital in the holistic journey to improved eyesight.

The Impact of Emotional States on Eyesight

1. **Stress and Vision**: Chronic stress results in the release of cortisol, the body's primary stress hormone. Elevated cortisol levels can increase intraocular pressure, potentially contributing to conditions like glaucoma. Moreover, stress can strain the tiny muscles around the eyes, leading to blurred vision and headaches.

2. **Anxiety and Hyper-Focus**: Individuals with anxiety often exhibit a hyper-focused gaze, where the peripheral vision narrows. This "tunnel vision" is a primal response, originally designed to help us focus on threats. Over time, persistent anxiety can limit our natural field of vision.

3. **Emotional Trauma and Blurred Vision**: In some instances,

traumatic events can lead to a sudden loss of vision, known as 'hysterical blindness'. Although the eyes are physically capable of seeing, the brain blocks out vision as a coping mechanism.

4. **Mood and Light Sensitivity**: Our emotional state can influence our sensitivity to light. Depression, for instance, has been linked to increased light sensitivity, where individuals may find bright environments overwhelming.

Fostering Emotional Balance for Vision Health

1. **Mindfulness Meditation**: This practice emphasizes staying present, acknowledging thoughts and feelings without judgment. Regular mindfulness meditation can reduce stress and anxiety, thereby benefiting vision. It also trains the eyes to relax, shifting focus effortlessly without straining.

2. **Deep Breathing Exercises**: Deep, diaphragmatic breathing can activate the body's relaxation response. When practiced regularly, it can help alleviate eye strain resulting from stress.

3. **Emotional Freedom Techniques (EFT)**: Sometimes referred to as 'tapping', EFT involves tapping on specific meridian points while voicing positive affirmations. This can help in releasing emotional blockages that may be affecting vision.

4. **Journaling**: Writing down feelings, fears, and frustrations can provide clarity and emotional release. Over time, it might reveal patterns or triggers adversely impacting one's emotional and visual health.

5. **Regular Counselling or Therapy**: Speaking with a professional can help address deeper emotional issues or traumas that might be influencing vision. They can offer coping techniques tailored to individual needs.

6. **Visualization Techniques**: Visualization or guided imagery can be an effective way to address anxiety. Imagining serene, expansive landscapes can train the eyes to relax and look into

the distance, countering the narrowing effect of anxiety.

7. **Nature Walks**: Nature has a calming effect on the psyche. Regular walks in nature can reduce stress and offer the eyes a refreshing break from screen-intensive environments. The natural landscapes provide opportunities to practice distant gazing and dynamic focusing.

8. **Yoga and Tai Chi**: These holistic practices combine movement with mindfulness. They help in reducing stress, improving posture, and increasing blood circulation, including to the eyes.

9. **Adequate Sleep**: Emotional well-being is closely tied to sleep quality. Ensure a restful night's sleep to give the eyes and the mind the rejuvenation they need.

10. **Limit Stimulants**: Excessive caffeine or sugar can exacerbate anxiety and stress. Moderation is key.

11. **Connect Socially**: Human connection is vital for emotional balance. Spending time with loved ones or engaging in group activities can uplift mood and provide emotional support.

Conclusion

Our vision is a complex interplay of physical and emotional factors. Just as the eyes need exercises and good habits to stay in optimal condition, our emotional health requires care and attention. By recognizing the profound influence our emotional states exert on our vision, we can adopt practices to ensure both our eyes and our psyche are nurtured. Emotional well-being is not merely about feeling good; it's an essential facet of the journey towards perfect sight without glasses.

CHAPTER 53: THE SCIENCE BEHIND "EYE YOGA"

Yoga, an ancient practice rooted in Indian philosophy, has transcended time and borders to become a global phenomenon. Its principles of balance, relaxation, and holistic wellness have found application in many spheres, including the realm of vision improvement. "Eye Yoga" emerges from the intersection of traditional yogic principles and modern understanding of visual health. Let's delve into the science and history behind this intriguing practice.

Understanding Eye Yoga: The Concept and Origins

At its core, yoga promotes the harmony of body, mind, and spirit. It encourages practitioners to develop mindfulness and physical flexibility. "Eye Yoga" borrows from these principles, focusing specifically on the muscles and health of the eyes.

Historically, yogic texts have always emphasized the importance of vision. For instance, 'Trataka', an ancient yogic practice, involves gazing at a single point, such as a candle flame, to enhance concentration and stimulate the eyes. This practice laid the foundation for what would later evolve into a broader discipline of eye-centric exercises.

The science behind "Eye Yoga" relies on the fact that our eyes have several muscles, which, like any other muscles in the body, can get strained or fatigued. Regularly exercising and relaxing these muscles can promote better vision and prevent degenerative issues.

Practical Eye Yoga Exercises

1. **Palming**: This technique is all about relaxing the eyes. Rub your hands together to generate warmth. Then, gently cup your eyes with your palms without putting pressure on the eyeballs. The darkness and warmth allow the eye muscles to relax. Breathe deeply and visualize a tranquil scene.

2. **Sideways Viewing**: Sit comfortably with legs straight in front of your body. Lift your arms, keeping them straight, to the side at shoulder height. With the thumbs pointing upwards, slowly move the eyes towards the left thumb, then towards the space between the eyebrows (third eye) and finally towards the right thumb. Repeat this for about 10-15 times, followed by closing the eyes and relaxing.

3. **Front and Sideways Viewing**: Keeping your neck stationary, look straight ahead. Without moving your head, direct your gaze as far to the left as possible, and then as far to the right. Return to the central point, and then look as high and as low as you can. Repeat several times, and then relax your eyes.

4. **Rotational Viewing**: Sit upright with legs in front of you. Place the left hand on the left knee. Hold the right fist above the right knee, with the thumb pointing upwards and the elbow straight. Keep the head still, focus on the thumb, and make a circle with the thumb, keeping the elbows straight. Track the motion of the thumb with your eyes as it moves in both clockwise and counter clockwise directions.

5. **Near and Distant Viewing**: Stand or sit by a window with a clear view of the horizon. Focus on the tip of your nose for a moment, and then shift your focus to a distant object on the horizon. Alternate this near and distant focus several times

before closing and relaxing your eyes.

6. **Blinking**: Simple yet effective. Rapidly blink your eyes for a few seconds. Pause and then blink every 3-4 seconds for a minute or two. This exercise helps refresh the eyes and can prevent strain, especially for those who spend long hours in front of screens.

Benefits and Outcomes

"Eye Yoga" offers multiple benefits. Regular practice can enhance focus, reduce eye strain, and improve coordination between both eyes, leading to better depth perception and 3D vision. Additionally, these exercises stimulate the flow of essential nutrients and oxygen to the eyes, promoting overall eye health.

In Conclusion

While "Eye Yoga" cannot replace professional vision care or guarantee a reversal of severe vision issues, it offers a natural way to maintain and potentially enhance visual health. By incorporating these exercises into daily routines, we not only promote better vision but also embrace an age-old philosophy of balance and holistic well-being. As with any exercise regimen, consistency is key, and the benefits of "Eye Yoga" unfold most significantly with dedicated practice.

CHAPTER 54: VISION AND POSTURE: THE CONNECTION

We often think of vision as an isolated system, functioning independently from the rest of our body. In reality, our eyes are intricately connected to various bodily systems, with our posture playing a pivotal role in our visual health. The way we stand, sit, and carry ourselves can profoundly impact our eyesight. Let's explore this intriguing connection between vision and posture.

The Interrelation of Vision and Posture

Posture, at its essence, refers to the way we position our body while standing, sitting, or lying down. Proper posture ensures the alignment of the spine, promoting efficient bodily function and minimizing strain. When we adopt poor postural habits, it creates a cascade of physiological changes, some of which directly or indirectly affect our vision.

1. **Spinal Alignment and Eye Level**: A misaligned spine often leads to the head tilting forward or sideways. When our head isn't level, it changes the angle at which our eyes interact with our environment, straining the eye muscles and impacting visual accuracy.

2. **Blood Circulation**: Poor posture can impede optimal blood flow, depriving the eyes of essential nutrients and oxygen. This

can result in visual fatigue and reduce the eyes' ability to repair and regenerate.

3. **Neck Tension**: Holding the head in an unnatural position strains the neck muscles. These muscles have a network of nerves connected to the visual system. Tension here can trigger headaches, directly affecting visual comfort.

Tips for Good Posture

1. **Awareness**: Regularly check in with your body. Self-awareness is the first step in correcting postural habits. Pay attention to how you sit at your desk, stand in a queue, or even relax on a couch.

2. **Ergonomic Workspace**: If you work at a desk, ensure your workstation is set up to promote good posture. The computer screen should be at eye level, arms should form a 90-degree angle at the elbows, and feet should rest flat on the ground.

3. **Take Breaks**: When engrossed in work or a captivating book, we often forget to move. Set reminders to take short breaks every 30 minutes to stretch, walk around, and reset your posture.

4. **Core Strengthening**: A strong core supports spinal alignment. Incorporate exercises like planks, palates, or yoga into your routine to strengthen your abdominal muscles.

Exercises to Enhance Posture for Optimal Eyesight

1. **Chin Tucks**: This exercise strengthens the neck muscles and corrects forward head posture. Sit or stand tall. Without tilting your head, gently draw your chin backward, creating a double chin. Hold for 5 seconds, relax, and repeat.

2. **Wall Angels**: Stand with your back against a wall, feet shoulder-width apart. Your head, upper back, and lower back should touch the wall. Raise your arms to the sides, forming a 'W' shape, with the back of your hands against the wall. Slowly

slide your arms upwards, forming a 'Y' shape, and then return to the 'W'. Ensure your arms maintain contact with the wall throughout.

3. **Shoulder Blade Squeeze**: Sit or stand tall. Imagine holding a pencil between your shoulder blades and squeeze them together. Hold for a few seconds, then release.

4. **Thoracic Extension**: Sit tall in a chair. Place your hands behind your head, elbows pointing outward. Gently arch your upper back while looking slightly upwards. Hold for a few seconds, then return to the starting position.

5. **Text Neck Correction**: If you're often looking down at your phone, practice lifting it to eye level. This small change can significantly reduce neck and eye strain.

In Conclusion

Our bodies function as an interconnected system. The relationship between posture and vision underscores the importance of holistic well-being. When we prioritize good posture, we're not just safeguarding our spine but also promoting optimal visual health. Remember, every time you stand tall, sit straight, or adjust your workspace, you're taking a step toward clearer, more comfortable vision.

CHAPTER 55: EXPLORING VISION SUPPLEMENTS: FACTS AND MYTHS

In our quest for optimal vision health, many of us have encountered numerous supplements that claim to enhance or maintain our eyesight. With so many options available, how can we discern fact from fiction? This chapter delves into some of the most popular vision supplements, examining the science behind them, and providing an informed perspective on their use.

Popular Supplements for Eye Health

1. **Lutein and Zeaxanthin**: These carotenoids, found naturally in the retina, play a crucial role in protecting the eyes from harmful high-energy light waves like ultraviolet rays. Their antioxidant properties defend the eyes from oxidative damage, which can lead to conditions like age-related macular degeneration (AMD) and cataracts.

   * **Scientific Evidence**: Numerous studies have showcased the protective qualities of these carotenoids. For instance, the AREDS2 (Age-Related Eye Disease Study 2) demonstrated that participants with higher dietary intake of lutein and zeaxanthin had a reduced risk of developing advanced AMD.

* **Recommended Dosage**: While there's no established daily recommendation, many studies have utilized 10 mg of lutein and 2 mg of zeaxanthin daily.

2. **Omega-3 Fatty Acids**: Commonly found in fish oils, these fatty acids are essential for maintaining the fluidity of cell membranes in the eyes. They also have anti-inflammatory properties that can combat conditions like dry eyes.

* **Scientific Evidence**: Multiple studies indicate that omega-3 supplements can help reduce symptoms of dry eye, enhancing tear production and reducing eye inflammation.

* **Recommended Dosage**: Dosages vary, but many studies suggest benefits with intakes of 1000-1200 mg daily.

3. **Vitamin C**: An antioxidant, vitamin C helps maintain the health of blood vessels in the eyes and may protect against cataract development.

* **Scientific Evidence**: Observational studies have linked high vitamin C intake with reduced risk of cataracts. Moreover, vitamin C, when combined with other antioxidants, was found in the AREDS study to reduce the progression of AMD.

* **Recommended Dosage**: A typical daily dose for eye health ranges between 250-500 mg, but it's crucial to consult with a healthcare provider, as high doses can cause side effects.

4. **Zinc**: This essential trace mineral plays a vital role in transporting vitamin A from the liver to the retina, aiding in melanin production.

* **Scientific Evidence**: The original AREDS study found that zinc supplementation, especially when combined with antioxidants, reduced the risk of developing advanced AMD.

* **Recommended Dosage**: The AREDS study used 80 mg of zinc oxide, but this dosage can lead to side effects. It's

vital to discuss with a healthcare professional before starting supplementation.

Myths and Cautions

While supplements can offer benefits, it's essential to approach them with a discerning eye:

1. **Natural Intake is Best**: Obtaining nutrients from whole foods ensures balanced intake and offers additional beneficial compounds not found in supplements.
2. **Avoid Over-supplementation**: More doesn't always mean better. High doses can lead to adverse effects and interact with other medications.
3. **One Size Doesn't Fit All**: Everyone's nutritional needs and health conditions vary. What works for one person might not work for another.

In Conclusion

Supplementation can be a beneficial part of an eye health regimen, but it's not a substitute for a balanced diet, proper eye care, and regular check-ups. Before starting any new supplement, always consult with a healthcare professional or eye specialist to ensure it's the right choice for you.

Armed with knowledge, we can make informed decisions that prioritize the health and longevity of our vision, separating the facts from the myths in the world of vision supplements.

CHAPTER 56: BLUE LIGHT: ITS EFFECTS AND HOW TO PROTECT AGAINST IT

In our modern digital age, blue light exposure has become a hot topic, both for its potential benefits and its possible drawbacks. From smartphones to LED bulbs, the omnipresence of blue light sources is undeniable. But what does this mean for our eyes? Let's delve deeper into understanding blue light, its impact on our vision, and ways we can safeguard our eyes.

Understanding Blue Light

Blue light is part of the visible light spectrum, with a wavelength between 380 nm and 500 nm. Due to its short wavelength, blue light scatters more easily than other visible light, which is why the sky appears blue on a sunny day. While the primary source of blue light is sunlight, digital screens (like computers and smartphones), LED lighting, and fluorescent lights also emit a significant amount.

Impacts of Blue Light

1. **Circadian Rhythm and Sleep**: Blue light plays a pivotal role in regulating our body's internal clock or circadian rhythm. Exposure to blue light during daytime hours can boost attention, reaction times, and mood. However,

excessive exposure during the evening can suppress melatonin production, potentially disrupting sleep patterns.

2. **Eye Strain and Discomfort**: Digital Eye Strain, sometimes referred to as Computer Vision Syndrome, can be exacerbated by prolonged exposure to screen-emitted blue light. Symptoms include dry eyes, headache, blurred vision, and difficulty focusing.

3. **Potential Retinal Damage**: Some research suggests that prolonged exposure to blue light might lead to damaged retinal cells, potentially leading to age-related macular degeneration (AMD). However, conclusive evidence is still pending.

Reducing Blue Light Exposure

1. **Follow the 20-20-20 Rule**: To reduce eye strain, every 20 minutes, take a 20-second break and focus on something 20 feet away. This simple rule helps in giving the eyes a short period of rest, reducing the prolonged effects of staring at screens.

2. **Adjust Screen Settings**: Many devices come with a "night mode" or "warm colour" setting that reduces blue light emission. Activating this feature, especially during the evening, can help in reducing its potential impact on sleep.

3. **Ambient Lighting**: Ensure the room lighting is balanced. If the screen appears as a light source in the room, it might be too bright. Conversely, if it seems dull and gray, it might be too dark.

Protective Tools Against Blue Light

1. **Blue-light-blocking Glasses**: These are specialized eyeglasses that have filters in their lenses that block or absorb blue light from getting through. While they can be beneficial for those spending extensive hours in front of screens, it's essential to choose a quality pair that has been scientifically tested.

2. **Screen Filters**: Available for smartphones, tablets, and computer screens, these filters can prevent a significant amount

of blue light emission from reaching the eyes without affecting the visibility of the display.

3. **Anti-reflective Lenses**: For those who wear prescription glasses, lenses with anti-reflective coating can reduce blue light exposure, especially if you're under LED or fluorescent lights often.

In Conclusion

While the modern world has made screens and artificial lighting a central part of our lives, awareness and moderation are keys. By understanding the potential impacts of blue light and adopting practices to reduce excessive exposure, we can enjoy the benefits of technology without compromising our visual health.

It's crucial to remember that while blue light from screens is a concern, the most substantial exposure comes from the sun. So, while it's beneficial to be cautious of our screen time, it's equally vital to protect our eyes outdoors with sunglasses that block both UV and blue light.

In the journey towards perfect sight, recognizing and navigating the challenges of our digital age is imperative. With knowledge, protective tools, and mindful habits, we can ensure that our vision remains sharp and our eyes healthy amidst a sea of screens.

CHAPTER 57: THE ROLE OF SLEEP IN VISION HEALTH

Sleep is nature's way of rejuvenating the body, refreshing the mind, and, significantly, repairing our eyes. When we think about maintaining good eyesight, elements like diet, exercise, and protective measures often come to the forefront. However, the often overlooked, yet immensely crucial aspect, is the quality and quantity of our sleep. This chapter delves into the symbiotic relationship between sleep and vision health and offers tips to ensure our eyes reap the full benefits of restful nights.

The Eye During Wakefulness and Sleep

During waking hours, our eyes are in a state of constant activity – adjusting to various light intensities, focusing on different distances, and processing a plethora of visual information. By the end of the day, just like an overworked muscle, the eye too needs its downtime.

When we sleep, our eyes aren't just idly resting. They are undergoing a series of essential restorative processes:
1. **Cell Repair and Regeneration**: The eyes, especially the cornea, undergo vital repair and regeneration processes during sleep. Without adequate sleep, this repair can remain incomplete, leading to potential visual issues and discomfort.

2. **Tear Secretion and Eye Cleaning**: During sleep, the reduced tear production allows for a balanced tear film on the eyes. Also, beneficial tears are secreted during the deep stages of sleep that help remove waste products and debris.

3. **Nutrient Supply**: The state of rest facilitates the efficient supply of nutrients to the eye, ensuring it's well-nourished and ready for the next day's challenges.

Impact of Sleep Deprivation on Eyesight

Inconsistent or poor sleep can lead to several eye-related issues:
1. **Dry Eyes**: Lack of sleep can reduce the eye's ability to produce tears, leading to dry and itchy eyes.

2. **Twitching**: Ever noticed an involuntary eyelid spasm after a sleepless night? That's an eye twitch, often a result of fatigue.

3. **Blurry Vision**: Prolonged wakefulness can strain the eye muscles, leading to temporary blurriness.

4. **Increased Sensitivity**: Sleep-deprived eyes can become more sensitive to light, causing discomfort in bright environments.

5. **Reduced Focus**: The eye's ability to focus can be compromised, leading to difficulty in reading or performing close-up tasks.

Ensuring Quality Sleep for Optimal Eye Health

Given the critical role of sleep-in vision health, ensuring consistent, quality rest becomes paramount. Here are some actionable tips to cultivate better sleep habits:

1. **Consistency is Key**: Try to sleep and wake up at the same time every day. Regular sleep patterns can set your internal clock and improve the quality of your sleep.

2. **Create a Restful Environment**: Ensure your bedroom is

dark, quiet, and cool. Consider using earplugs, an eye mask, or a white-noise machine if needed.

3. **Limit Screen Time Before Bed**: The blue light from screens can interfere with melatonin production, making it harder to fall asleep. Aim to disconnect from screens at least an hour before bedtime.

4. **Mind Your Diet**: Avoid large meals, caffeine, and alcohol before bed. These can disrupt sleep and reduce its restorative quality.

5. **Incorporate Relaxation Techniques**: Consider adding practices like reading, meditation, or deep-breathing exercises to your bedtime routine. These can prepare the mind for restful sleep.

6. **Seek Professional Advice**: If you suffer from chronic insomnia or other sleep disorders, consulting a sleep specialist can provide tailored strategies and interventions.

In Conclusion

Our eyes, the windows to our soul, work tirelessly throughout the day to provide us with the gift of sight. And just like any other part of our body, they require adequate rest to function optimally. Recognizing the vital role of sleep in maintaining and improving vision can propel us towards habits that honour both our need for rest and our desire for perfect sight.

In our journey to natural vision improvement, let us remember that sometimes the best remedy is the simplest one – a good night's sleep. Through rest, repair, and rejuvenation, our eyes will be better equipped to serve us each new day.

Part VI: Real-Life Success Stories

CHAPTER 58:
JANE'S JOURNEY

Jane Williams, a 32-year-old graphic designer, epitomizes the possibility of reclaiming one's vision naturally. Her journey from being tethered to a strong prescription to embracing the clarity of 20/20 vision is both heartening and instructive. This chapter charts Jane's odyssey, offering insights and inspirations to anyone on the path to natural vision improvement.

Discovering the Dependency

Jane first realized her vision was faltering during her high school years. Initially mistaking her blurry blackboard vision for fatigue, she soon found out, through a routine eye examination, that she had myopia. What began as a mild prescription for glasses quickly intensified as she entered college, and soon Jane was dependent on her spectacles for almost every waking moment.

With her profession as a graphic designer, she was spending prolonged hours in front of a computer screen, further straining her eyes. Her glasses became thicker, and her dependency on them became more pronounced with each passing year.

The Turning Point

It was during a vacation in the Maldives, amidst its crystal-clear waters and pristine beaches, that Jane felt the weight of her glasses most acutely. It pained her that she couldn't dive into the water without her prescription goggles or enjoy the sunset without the ever-present glare on her lenses.

While sharing her frustrations with a fellow traveller, she was introduced to the world of natural vision improvement. Sceptical but intrigued, Jane decided to research more upon her return.

Embarking on the Natural Path

Jane began by reading various books and attending seminars on natural vision improvement. The Bates Method, palming, sunning, and eye yoga were all new concepts to her. But, instead of feeling overwhelmed, she felt a burgeoning hope.

She started with simple practices:
1. **Regular Breaks**: Every 20 minutes of screen time, she'd gaze at a distant object for 20 seconds.
2. **Palming**: To relax her eye muscles, she'd cover her eyes with her palms a few times a day, feeling the warmth seep in.
3. **Sunning**: With closed eyes, she'd let the sun's rays gently warm her lids every morning.

Jane also enrolled in an eye yoga class, learning exercises that would enhance her focus, flexibility, and overall eye health.

Challenges Along the Way

The path wasn't devoid of challenges. Initially, Jane was often met with scepticism from friends and even family. Many questioned her decision to reduce her screen time or take frequent breaks, especially given her profession.

But the most significant challenge was internal. On days when she felt there was no improvement, doubts clouded her resolve. She wondered if she was on a futile quest, whether she should accept her glasses as an unchangeable part of her life.

Seeing the Change

However, with time and consistent effort, the changes, though subtle at first, became more evident. Six months into her practices, during a routine eye check-up, her optometrist confirmed that her prescription had reduced.

Elated, Jane doubled down on her efforts. She also delved into the emotional aspects of vision, realizing that her eyesight was linked to her inner state. Meditation and mindfulness became part of her daily routine.

Achieving 20/20 Vision

Two years from the day she decided to embark on this journey, Jane achieved what she once deemed impossible - 20/20 vision. The thick glasses that were once a staple were now a relic of the past.

Her achievement wasn't just about the clarity of sight but also about the clarity of mind and the rejuvenated spirit with which she approached life.

Conclusion

Jane's journey is a testament to the power of determination, consistency, and belief. It showcases that with the right tools and mindset, our body's natural ability to heal and adapt can work wonders. Her story serves as an inspiration to all, reminding us that sometimes, the vision of a better future is all the motivation one needs to start.

CHAPTER 59: MARK'S MIRACLE

In the realm of vision stories, Mark Thompson's stands out as a beacon of hope for those battling astigmatism. Often deemed a condition relegated to the realm of surgical interventions or corrective lenses, Mark's experience showcases a different narrative. His miracle didn't arise from a surgeon's blade but from a melding of determination, patience, and natural techniques.

Understanding Astigmatism

Before delving into Mark's journey, it's crucial to understand astigmatism. Essentially, it's an imperfection in the curvature of one's cornea or lens. Instead of having a symmetrically rounded shape — like a basketball — the eye's surface might curve more in one direction than in another — more like a rugby ball. This causes light to be refracted unevenly, leading to blurred or distorted vision.

The Onset of Mark's Challenge

Mark first realized his vision was off kilter during his late twenties. Straight lines began to warp, and reading became a challenge. Night driving was especially taxing, with oncoming headlights appearing as elongated streaks.

Upon an eye examination, the verdict was clear: Mark had astigmatism. He was given a prescription for toric lenses, specially designed to counteract the irregular curvature of his eyes.

The Decision to Tread an Alternative Path

While the glasses offered a temporary solution, Mark was not content. The idea of being forever dependent on lenses, or potentially undergoing surgery, was daunting. He yearned for a natural resolution.

One evening, during a meditation session, Mark had an epiphany. If the body could heal cuts and broken bones, perhaps the eye, a much more sophisticated organ, also had the intrinsic power to mend itself. This thought was the genesis of his natural vision improvement pursuit.

Integrative Approaches and Techniques

Mark's first action step was to reduce his dependency on his glasses. He began to use them only when absolutely necessary. While this was initially challenging, it forced his eyes to work harder, potentially aiding in their natural recalibration.

He then dove deep into eye exercises that focused on strengthening the eye muscles and improving flexibility. Some of the techniques he embraced included:

1. **Pinhole Glasses**: These glasses, punctuated with multiple pin-sized holes, eliminate peripheral light and make the eyes focus on what's directly in front of them. This simple act can help reduce the irregular focusing caused by astigmatism.
2. **Focusing Exercises**: Mark would regularly practice shifting his focus from near to far objects, enhancing the eyes' focusing ability.
3. **Eye Rolling**: By slowly rolling his eyes in a circular motion, Mark aimed to improve the flexibility of his eye muscles.
4. **Visualization and Relaxation**: Understanding the mind-eye connection, Mark would often visualize his eyes' curvature returning to its ideal shape. Accompanied by deep breathing, this not only relaxed him but also set a powerful intention for

healing.

The Role of Holistic Wellness

In tandem with these exercises, Mark embarked on a holistic wellness journey. He improved his diet, incorporated vision-boosting foods, practiced yoga, and embraced mindfulness. All these seemingly unrelated practices contributed to his overall well-being, which in turn positively impacted his vision.

The Culmination: Mark's Miracle

About a year and a half into his natural vision improvement regimen, Mark scheduled an eye examination. The result was nothing short of miraculous. His astigmatism had considerably reduced. While not entirely gone, the change was significant enough that he no longer needed his glasses.

Emboldened, Mark continued his practices. Another year passed, and a subsequent check-up revealed the unimaginable — his eyes were nearly perfect. The astigmatism had corrected itself to a point where it was almost negligible.

In Retrospect

Mark's journey underscores that while each person's body and circumstances are unique, there's undeniable power in natural processes and the body's innate ability to heal. His story serves as an inspiration, demonstrating that with dedication, belief, and the right practices, overcoming challenges — even astigmatism without surgery — is within the realm of possibility.

CHAPTER 60:
THE FUTURE OF
NATURAL VISION
IMPROVEMENT

Where Science Meets Holistic Approaches

As we conclude our journey through the avenues of natural vision improvement, it's crucial to glance forward and discern what the future holds for this realm. The integration of science and holistic methods is pushing the boundaries of what's achievable, offering hope to countless individuals worldwide. Here's a look into the intriguing nexus of science, technology, and ancient wisdom.

A Re-emphasis on Prevention

In the future, the focus will likely pivot even more towards prevention rather than correction. The adage "an ounce of prevention is worth a pound of cure" rings especially true for eye health. With the escalating concerns over screen time, blue light exposure, and modern lifestyle challenges, there's a pressing need to integrate preventive practices into daily routines. Proactive measures, from ergonomic adjustments to digital detox regimes, are expected to gain paramount importance.

Blending Technology with Tradition

While technology might seem like a culprit exacerbating vision issues, it also emerges as a potential ally. Already, we are witnessing apps that remind users to take breaks, ensure they blink regularly, or even guide them through eye exercises. Future technological advancements might utilize augmented reality or virtual reality to guide individuals through comprehensive vision therapy sessions, melding age-old techniques with modern innovation.

Holistic Wellness: A Comprehensive Approach

Science is beginning to understand the intricate links between overall well-being and specific facets of health, including vision. With this, there's a growing acknowledgment of the importance of mental health, emotional balance, diet, physical activity, and even spiritual wellness in maintaining and improving visual acuity. The future promises a more integrative approach, where eye health isn't seen in isolation but as a part of the holistic health mosaic.

Research and Clinical Studies

As interest in natural vision improvement grows, so does the body of research surrounding it. Scientists are investigating everything from the efficacy of specific eye exercises to the impact of dietary supplements on vision health. As more empirical data emerges, it will solidify the foundation of natural vision improvement, offering clear protocols backed by science.

Bridging the Gap: Collaboration between Optometrists and Holistic Practitioners

Historically, there's been a divide between mainstream optometrists and proponents of natural vision techniques. The future promises a more collaborative approach. It's easy to foresee a world where an optometrist's office doesn't just stop at prescribing glasses or contact lenses but extends its services to include sessions on eye yoga, recommendations on vision-boosting foods, or even meditation classes for visual relaxation.

Customized Approaches

The recognition that every individual is unique will underscore the importance of personalization. Just as today's medicine is gradually moving towards personalized treatments based on genetic makeup and individual health profiles, the realm of vision care will evolve to provide bespoke solutions. Factors such as one's lifestyle, work environment, genetic predispositions, and personal preferences will play a role in shaping individualized vision care plans.

In Conclusion

The journey of "Perfect Sight Without Glasses" has been an exploration of the harmonious blend of ancient wisdom and modern science. It emphasizes that while external aids like glasses and surgeries have their place, the body's intrinsic capacity to heal, adapt, and improve cannot be side-lined.

As we stand on the cusp of exciting breakthroughs and approaches in vision care, it becomes evident that the future of natural vision improvement is bright, promising, and incredibly empowering. The key lies in being open-minded, proactive, and always ready to embrace the synergy of science and holistic health.

Your vision is a precious gift, and as you move forward, may you harness the vast reservoir of natural techniques, informed choices, and scientific advances to cherish, protect, and enhance this invaluable treasure.

Appendices

A. Suggested Reading and Resources

1. **Books**:
   - "The Art of Seeing" by Aldous Huxley: A personal narrative

detailing Huxley's own experiences with natural vision improvement.

- "Better Eyesight Without Glasses" by William H. Bates: The seminal work that introduced many of the techniques discussed in this guide.

- "Take Off Your Glasses and See" by Jacob Liberman: A holistic approach to reclaiming perfect sight.

2. **Websites**:

- [EyeExercise.org] (#): Comprehensive site offering a variety of exercises and techniques.

- [NaturalVisionForum.net] (#): An active community of individuals sharing personal experiences, challenges, and success stories.

3. **Mobile Apps**:

- **Eye Relax**: Reminds you to take breaks and guides through relaxation techniques.

- **Vision Trainer**: Offers a range of exercises to improve eye strength and focus.

B. Daily and Weekly Vision Improvement Routines

Daily Routine:
1. **Morning Palming** (5 minutes): Upon waking up, rub your hands together until warm, then gently cup them over your eyes. Feel the warmth seeping in, relaxing your eye muscles.
2. **Blinking Exercise** (2 minutes): Ensure that you blink regularly, especially if working on screens. Aim to blink consciously every 3-4 seconds for a couple of minutes.
3. **Near-Far Focus** (5 minutes): This exercise can be incorporated during work breaks. Shift focus from a close object (e.g., your finger) to a distant one, alternating every few seconds.
4. **Eye Rolls** (3 minutes): Slowly roll your eyes in a clockwise and then counter clockwise direction. Helps in maintaining flexibility.

Weekly Routine:
1. **Nature Walks** (30 minutes, twice a week): Spend time in nature, focusing on distant objects, varying landscapes, and natural colours.
2. **Screen-Free Saturdays**: Dedicate one day a week to drastically reduce screen time. Engage in hobbies, physical activities, or simply relax.
3. **Dietary Check**: Ensure weekly consumption of foods rich in Vitamin A, omega-3 fatty acids, and antioxidants. Consider carrots, spinach, fatty fish, and berries.
4. **Meditation and Relaxation** (20 minutes, 3 times a week): Focus on calming the mind, which indirectly aids visual relaxation.

C. Glossary of Terms

- **Accommodation**: The ability of the eye to change its focus from distant to near objects (and vice versa). This process is achieved by the lens changing its shape.

- **Amblyopia**: Often referred to as "lazy eye," it's a vision developmental disorder where one eye fails to achieve normal visual acuity, even with prescription glasses or contact lenses.

- **Astigmatism**: A common vision condition that causes blurred vision due to either the irregular shape of the cornea or sometimes the curvature of the lens inside the eye.

- **Bates Method**: A natural vision improvement technique developed by Dr. William H. Bates in the early 20th century. It involves a series of exercises to train the eyes to focus correctly.

- **Binocular Vision**: The ability to maintain visual focus on an object with both eyes, creating a single visual image.

- **Cones**: Photoreceptor cells in the retina responsible for colour vision.

- **Palming**: A relaxation technique where the palms are rubbed together to produce warmth and then placed gently over the eyes.

- **Presbyopia**: A natural condition where, as age progresses, the eye exhibits a progressively diminished ability to focus on near objects.

- **Rods**: Photoreceptor cells in the retina responsible for vision in low light conditions.

Incorporating the aforementioned routines, understanding the glossary, and diving deeper with the recommended resources will further enhance your journey towards perfect sight without glasses.

D. Recommended Equipment and Tools

1. **Pinhole Glasses**: These glasses contain a series of pin-sized perforations, helping the eyes to focus and can be used for certain exercises.

2. **Eye Charts**: A standard Snellen eye chart can be placed in your home or office. Regularly practicing reading from varying distances can be beneficial.

3. **Blue Light Blocking Glasses**: If you spend considerable time in front of screens, these glasses can reduce eye strain by filtering out blue light emitted from digital devices.

4. **Eye Patches**: Useful for certain exercises aimed at strengthening a weaker eye, especially in cases of amblyopia or 'lazy eye'.

5. **Swing String**: A simple string with beads that can be used for the "Bead String Exercise" to improve convergence and depth perception.

E. Online Courses and Workshops

There are several online platforms offering courses on natural vision improvement. Some popular options include:

1. **The Bates Method International**: A comprehensive online course designed to teach the fundamentals of Dr. Bates' techniques.
2. **Natural Vision Academy**: This platform offers a variety of courses, from beginner to advanced, catering to different vision needs.
3. **Holistic Vision Summit**: An annual online event where leading experts in the field share their knowledge, techniques, and experiences.

F. Tips for Choosing a Vision Therapist

If you decide to seek professional guidance, consider these factors:

1. **Credentials**: Ensure the therapist has formal training and is certified by a recognized organization.
2. **Experience**: Look for therapists with a track record in helping individuals achieve tangible results.
3. **Approach**: The best therapists often combine traditional methods with holistic approaches, offering a comprehensive treatment plan.
4. **Referrals**: Ask for testimonials or referrals from past clients to gauge their satisfaction levels.

G. Quick Reference Guide to Exercises

For easy recall:

1. **Palming** - To relax the eyes.
2. **Blinking** - To moisten and give eyes a quick rest.
3. **Near-Far Focus** - To improve flexibility in accommodating different distances.
4. **Eye Rolls** - To enhance muscle flexibility.

5. **The Swing** - To improve motion detection and peripheral vision.

The journey to natural vision improvement is multi-faceted and enriched by a combination of knowledge, practice, and perseverance. These appendices are curated to be your constant companions, offering direction and clarity as you tread the path to perfect sight without glasses. Remember, the vision is not just about seeing the world but truly experiencing its beauty and depth.

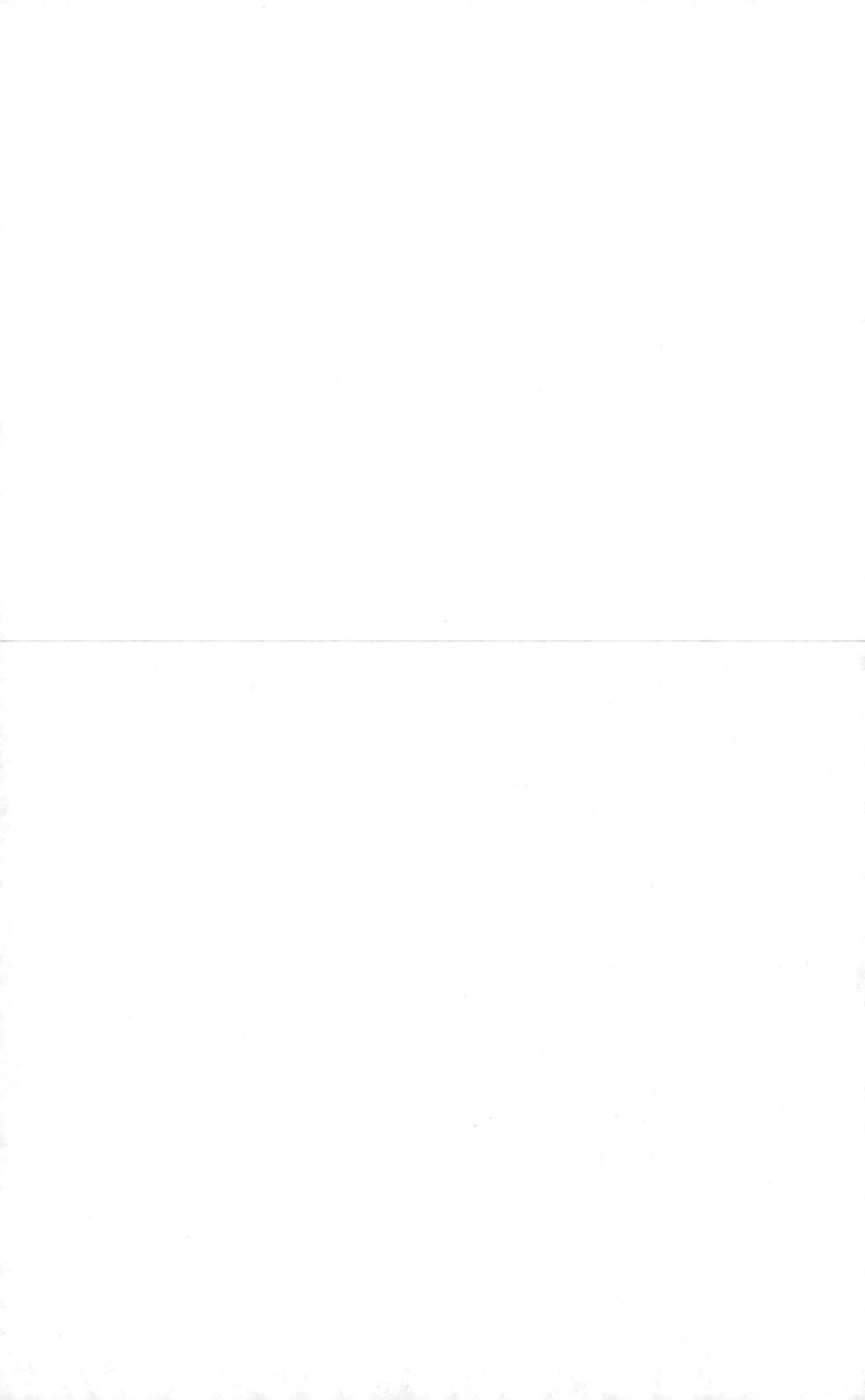